ALL ABOUT DRUGS AND DOCTORS

PREVENTION'S

FAMILY HEALTH LIBRARY™

ALL ABOUT DRUGS AND DOCTORS

A Consumer's Guide to Safe, Effective Medical Care

by the Editors of
Prevention® Magazine

 Rodale Press, Emmaus, Pa.

Copyright © 1987 by Rodale Press, Inc.

Printed in the United States of America on recycled paper containing a high percentage of de-inked fiber.

Library of Congress Cataloging in Publication Data

All about drugs and doctors.

    (Prevention's family health library)
    1. Medical economics. 2. Drugs. 3. Consumer education.   I. Prevention
(Emmaus, Pa.)   II. Series.
RA410.5.A45 1987   610   86-29854
ISBN 0-87857-705-X paperback

2 4 6 8 10 9 7 5 3 1 paperback

NOTICE

This book is intended as a reference volume only, not as a medical manual or guide to self-treatment. If you suspect that you have a medical problem, we urge you to seek competent medical help. Keep in mind that nutritional and health needs vary from person to person, depending on age, sex, health status and total diet. The information here is intended to help you make informed decisions about your health, not as a substitute for any treatment that may have been prescribed by your doctor.

Contents

CHAPTER 1

All about Aspirin and Its Substitutes

"Take two aspirin and call me in the morning." How many times have you heard that old saw? It's probably been around as long as aspirin itself. Thing is, while the saying hasn't changed over the years, the product's image certainly has. Along with plain aspirin, there's now extra-strength, arthritis-strength and maximum-strength aspirin (which basically give you more milligrams of aspirin per tablet), not to mention those combined with caffeine and buffers or the timed-release and coated varieties.

Then again, if the doctor's really with the times, he may be just as likely to say, "Take two *Tylenol* and call me in the morning." What he really means, of course, is acetaminophen, the generic mouthful that's recently been dubbed "nonaspirin" by other drug companies hoping to cut into the Tylenol market.

Over-the-counter pain relievers are *big* business, whether it's aspirin or acetaminophen. Literally billions of tablets are swallowed each year in an attempt to alleviate common, everyday aches and pains, and to reduce fevers of colds and flu. But the most important reason that these over-the-counter products continue to be the most widely used in the world is that they work—and work well.

"Both aspirin and acetaminophen do a great job of relieving pain and reducing fever," says Gary C. Cupit, Pharm.D., clinical associate professor of pharmacy at the Philadelphia College of Pharmacy and Science. "Just a regular dose of aspirin (650 milligrams, or two tablets) or a similar dose of acetaminophen has been shown over and over again in clinical tests to effectively reduce pain and fever."

Best for Inflammation

For some types of headaches, however, a smaller dose of aspirin can actually work better than a larger dose of acetaminophen. "The reason the smaller dose of aspirin is as effective, or more so, than the larger acetaminophen dose is unclear," says Bruce H. Peters, M.D., of Colorado Springs, Colorado. "But headache pain commonly has some throbbing component, suggesting that a sterile inflammation is a part of most headache pain. Aspirin has much stronger anti-inflammatory action than acetaminophen and thus, in headache pain, seems to exceed acetaminophen's action on a weight-for-weight basis."

In fact, it's aspirin's anti-inflammatory properties that makes it the drug doctors usually recommend when it comes to arthritis pain. Rheumatoid arthritis, that is. That's the form that's often accompanied by severe inflammation.

Osteoarthritis, on the other hand, is a result of wear and tear on the joints, and inflammation is usually mild or absent altogether. With osteoarthritis, either acetaminophen or aspirin can be equally effective. But not equally risk-free. With chronic conditions such as arthritis, where aspirin (or acetaminophen) use can be long term, the risk of side effects cannot be overlooked. In that department aspirin is the leader with gastrointestinal (GI) problems.

"Between 2 and 6 percent of patients [taking aspirin] will have dyspepsia [stomach discomfort], nausea and vomiting, while the loss of blood in the stools may be 10 to 20 times greater than normal, depending on the dose," doctors reported in the *British Medical Journal* (January 10, 1981).

The dose and duration are the keys. "Epidemiological evidence suggests that only persons who take aspirin regularly (on four or more days a week) or in large doses (more than 15 tablets a week) are likely to suffer acute gastrointestinal bleeding or gastric ulceration."

"The rate is much lower for occasional use," adds Dr. Cupit. "Less than 1 percent, in fact."

Even though aspirin lands in the stomach, that's not the only place it can cause bleeding. Nosebleeds that start without any obvious cause could be related to aspirin ingestion. So can heavy menstrual periods when aspirin is taken to prevent cramping. That's because aspirin is a potent platelet-aggregation inhibitor. (Platelets are tiny cells that help the blood clot.) A single aspirin tablet taken by a normal person can cause a "definite prolongation of the bleeding time" [a test which measures how quickly blood clots], says a researcher from Sweden. "A simple dose of 650 milligrams of aspirin [two regular-strength tablets] approximately doubles the mean bleeding time for a period of four to seven days" (*Pharmacy International,* October, 1982).

Nevertheless, some doctors think that *that* side effect isn't all bad either. Recent studies have suggested that aspirin's blood-thinning abilities may actually reduce the risk of heart attacks and strokes and may also be more helpful than sometimes thought in the prevention and treatment of migraine headaches.

While claims like those cannot be made for acetaminophen, this remedy *can* boast about its low incidence of side effects. At normal, recommended doses there's virtually nothing to report. "This is one of the safest drugs on the market," says Dr. Cupit. "Only rare cases of liver disease have been documented and those were usually associated with excessive use. That means more than four grams (eight extra-strength tablets) a day."

Unlike aspirin, there are no stomach upsets and no bleeding problems connected with acetaminophen—which accounts for its increasing popularity among doctors.

Which to Use?

From the look of it, the question of aspirin or acetaminophen is not really either/or—but when. Depending on what ails you, whether it's transient or chronic, what your general state of health is, and what (if any) other medications you're on, there are some specific guidelines you can follow to give you the best results with a minimum of risk.

• If you have any stomach disorders or ulcers, any medication containing aspirin should be avoided.

• To help reduce the chance of even mild stomach irritation, always take aspirin with a full glass of liquid.

• People with iron-deficiency anemia (common in the elderly) should avoid aspirin and use acetaminophen instead, because it does not cause any blood loss as aspirin may.

• Anyone preparing for surgery (even tooth extraction) should avoid aspirin at least a week or two before, because it can increase bleeding during the operation. Your doctor will probably recommend acetaminophen instead.

• For relief of chronic pain, first find out if you need the anti-inflammatory action of aspirin. If not, take acetaminophen. If inflammation *is* contributing to the problem (as in rheumatoid arthritis or certain muscular aches) take the newer enteric-coated or timed-release aspirin products. They may reduce the chances of gastric distress associated with aspirin, according to reports.

• In one study, researchers divided 20 healthy volunteers into four groups. They received either plain aspirin, buffered aspirin, enteric-coated aspirin or a placebo, three tablets administered four times a day for a total of seven days. Internal gastrointestinal examinations were done and pictures taken both before and again two hours after the medication period ended.

"Severe injury to the stomach and duodenum was found in all subjects taking buffered or plain aspirin," report the researchers. Except for one volunteer in the coated-aspirin group who had stomach injury, no others from this or the placebo group had any evidence of damage whatsoever (*New England Journal of Medicine,* July, 1980).

Designed to Bypass Stomach

• "The enteric-coated aspirin tablets are designed to dissolve in the small intestine," explains Dr. Cupit, "bypassing the stomach, where irritation usually occurs. As for the timed- or steady-release products, they are formulated to be pH-dependent. That means that the aspirin is not released until the tablet reaches the alkaline environment of the small intestine.

"With either of these products, pain relief obviously will be delayed since they take longer to dissolve. That's okay for a chronic-pain situation where speed of onset is less important than maximum stomach protection. But they are not recommended for acute, short-term pain.

    • Conditions of acute or severe, transient pain such as headache or toothache require a quick-acting medication. Your choices are aspirin, acetaminophen (both in various strengths), buffered aspirin (tablets or solutions) or combination drugs. We already know that all these products work to relieve pain, but some work better than others. Let's start with combination drugs. Ever wonder why some of these products contain caffeine? Researchers have found that adding this substance, commonly found in coffee, actually enhances the painkilling effectiveness of the drug.

    • In one study, researchers compared the effectiveness of acetaminophen alone or in combination with 65 milligrams of caffeine. The 173 patients in the study had all had a molar extracted. The results showed that relief of pain was greater in the acetaminophen-plus-caffeine group than with acetaminophen alone. What's more, say the researchers, "the addition of caffeine to acetaminophen significantly shortened" the time it took for the drug to work (*Clinical Pharmacology and Therapeutics,* vol. 33, no. 4, 1983).

    • Other studies have shown that the same effect holds true when aspirin is combined with caffeine, too. The hitch is that it takes at least 60 milligrams of caffeine to get this enhanced painkilling effect, and most of the combination drugs (there are some exceptions) contain 30 milligrams or less. Also, you should remember that caffeine can be addicting, and the main withdrawal symptom on discontinuing caffeine is—you guessed it—a headache.

Some products combine acetaminophen with aspirin in the same tablet. But there's no evidence, according to researchers, that this is any more effective than either of these drugs alone.

What about Buffered?

    • As for buffered aspirin tablets, it's true that they dissolve faster—at least in a test tube—but there's no proof that they relieve pain faster in people. Nor is buffered aspirin gentler on the stomach than plain aspirin.

On the other hand, buffered aspirin solutions that you drink do cause less GI bleeding and may work faster since the drug is already dissolved. But these products have a high sodium content and are therefore not suitable for long-term use.

• Aspirin and acetaminophen are so commonplace in our lives that it's easy to forget that they are still drugs. And as such they must not be taken with certain other medications. Always tell your doctor if you are taking aspirin or acetaminophen on a regular basis when he is prescribing other medications.

Some drugs shouldn't be mixed with even *one* tablet of aspirin. In that category are alcohol (acetaminophen applies here, too), antacids, anticoagulants, antidiabetic drugs, corticosteroids, heparin and gout medications such as probenecid and sulfinpyrazone.

• Also, get in the habit of reading labels and talking to your pharmacist. Sometimes aspirin shows up where you least expect it, in prescription preparations as well as other over-the-counter products (allergy and cold remedies, for example).

• When it comes to giving these medicines to children, doctors are increasingly recommending acetaminophen. That's especially true for fever from viral infections. Studies have shown that children receiving aspirin during such illnesses have a greater chance of developing Reye's syndrome, a sometimes fatal complication of a minor viral infection (*Journal of the American Medical Association,* June 11, 1982).

• Remember that more is not necessarily better (and can be downright dangerous), even when it comes to drugs considered to be among the safest. Doctors suggest that you not exceed the recommended dosages on the packages (not more than four grams per day of either drug). If your symptoms are not relieved by this amount of medication, you need to see a doctor to determine if additional treatment is needed.

• Cost varies greatly among these products, but the most expensive brand names do not necessarily guarantee you a better product than the cheaper generic ones. As for those extra-strength, maximum-strength and arthritis-strength products—they give you more milligrams of medication per tablet but at a higher price. You could save money if you bought the plain aspirin or acetaminophen and simply took more tablets to equal the higher dosage. There is one benefit, though, for people who have trouble swallowing pills: They need fewer of the extra-strength variety.

Acetaminophen generally costs more than aspirin and the coated and timed-release varieties cost more, too. The newest form—capsule—offers no other benefit than being easier to swallow—but not after you see the price. That goes for those buffered solutions, as well.

• Never buy more pills than you can use in about a year, since these drugs lose potency and start to break down with time. Also, store your medications in a cool, dry place. The bathroom is probably the worst room in the house since the heat and humidity accelerate decomposition. If your aspirin starts to smell like vinegar, you'll know that it has deteriorated beyond usefulness.

Where Did They Come From?

If you think aspirin was invented in a laboratory by some ingenious scientist, you're in for a big surprise. In fact, aspirin is actually the modern variation of a very old folk remedy and it has been around much longer than any of us.

Ancient Romans, as well as American Indians, knew that they could reduce fever and pain by eating the bark of the willow tree. What they *didn't* know was that this tree bark contained the substance salicin, the forerunner of acetylsalicylic acid—or aspirin, as we know it today.

Although salicin is a very effective painkiller, it can be quite irritating to the stomach. So, scientists continued to refine the product and by the 1890's they had come up with acetylsalicylic acid—a combination of salicylic acid and acetic anhydride. Today, the herbal origins of aspirin are largely forgotten, although the Latin name for willows, *Salix,* remains a subtle reminder in the term acetyl*salic*ylic acid.

Acetaminophen is no newcomer to the drug scene, either. Surprised? It was actually discovered by accident in 1882 when a pharmacist incorrectly filled a prescription for two doctors who were treating a patient with intestinal parasites. The "wrong" medicine unexpectedly brought the patient's high fever down in a flash.

(continued)

Where Did They Come From? —*continued*

Upon investigating, the doctors found that they had given their patient a chemical called acetanilide. But it wasn't until 1899 that a German scientist discovered that acetanilide is metabolized in the body to become acetaminophen—the popular present-day "nonaspirin."

While the discovery is old, its surge in popularity is indeed recent. For no apparent reason acetaminophen did not spark the flurry of interest that aspirin had at the very same time. In fact, it wasn't until about 1950 that scientists in the United States began to examine its potential as an effective pain and fever reducer— and probably only then because English scientists had already confirmed its safety and effectiveness in their own clinical studies.

Today acetaminophen is the most rapidly growing part of the painreliever market.

CHAPTER 2

All about Digestive Aids

Heartburn. Gas. Acid stomach. Ulcer pain. It reaches the point where you don't care how you spell relief—as long as you get it, and fast.

For the millions of Americans who suffer from the burning aches and pains of digestive problems, there are hundreds of products that can bring relief—primarily by neutralizing stomach acid.

Everybody has stomach acid. You wouldn't be able to digest your food without it. Problems come up when it feels like the acid is digesting your stomach along with the food. With ulcers, that's just about the case. Since there's a break in the protective lining of the stomach, the acid is able to penetrate, causing the characteristic pain that usually accompanies ulcers.

But by far the most common use of antacids is for relief of *reflux esophagitis*—more commonly known as heartburn, acid indigestion or sour stomach. In these cases, the burning sensation doesn't usually take place in the stomach at all, but higher up, in the esophagus.

Normally, the stomach's contents are kept in the stomach and out of the esophagus by a special muscle, or sphincter, located between the two organs. But sometimes that muscle relaxes when it shouldn't, resulting in a reflux, or backing up, of the acidic juices. The lining of the esophagus is much more sensitive than the lining of the stomach, and it lets you know it by causing the uncomfortable burning sensation.

Antacids simply help neutralize the contents of the stomach so that the refluxed juices are no longer irritating. They don't neutralize all of the acid, but that really isn't necessary for the relief of pain.

Antacids also increase esophageal sphincter muscle tone, and that action may add to their effectiveness in heartburn relief.

There's no doubt that antacids are truly effective. Ask any heartburn sufferer who's just swallowed an antacid. Scientists have confirmed their usefulness, too. In one study, 33 heartburn sufferers were given either an antacid or placebo (harmless blank pill) for one month. Twenty-nine of the 33 correctly identified the antacid product, suggesting that the relief offered was not a placebo effect, say the researchers.

As for ulcers, antacids have been shown in clinical studies to not only relieve the symptoms but to actually promote healing as well. As one doctor has said, "No acid, no ulcer"—and apparently he was right.

Still, all antacids are not created equal, even if the end result is the same. Here's why. Antacid products contain at least one of four primary neutralizing ingredients: sodium bicarbonate, calcium carbonate, magnesium hydroxide and/or aluminum hydroxide, all of which you'll find in a tablet or liquid base. For the most part, they pass through your system quietly, neutralizing the acid and putting a smile back on your face. But depending on how much you take, or what other underlying problems may also be present, there is the possibility of picking up some mild to possibly severe side effects along the way. A closer look at each of the four ingredients is needed to explain it all.

Sodium Bicarbonate

Sodium bicarbonate (Alka-Seltzer, Bromo Seltzer) is a potent, effective antacid and will relieve your symptoms of indigestion or heartburn. "Taken for occasional digestive discomfort (once a week or less) there's nothing to worry about. But it is definitely *not* recommended for more frequent use or for chronic conditions such as ulcers," says Nicola Giacona, Pharm.D., supervisor of the Drug Information Center at the University of Utah, in Salt Lake City. Just a look at the name tells you why—*sodium* bicarbonate. "This is ordinary baking soda and it's loaded with sodium. Besides, it's completely soluble in the stomach and readily absorbed into the bloodstream, so it can lead to sodium overload and serious disturbances in the acid base balance of the body.

"Anyone on a salt-restricted diet (especially for high blood pressure) should forget products with sodium bicarbonate completely," adds Dr. Giacona. For example, a two-tablet dose of Alka-Seltzer contains 552 milligrams of sodium, enough to upset a salt-restricted diet.

The same is true if you're susceptible to fluid retention, since excessive sodium is usually involved with that problem, too. "Fortunately," says Dr. Giacona, "most brands have taken the sodium out of their products or reduced it drastically."

Calcium Carbonate

Calcium carbonate (Tums, Titralac, Alka-2) is also an excellent acid neutralizer, besides being fast-acting and inexpensive. While it is safe in small doses, regular or heavy use (more than six doses weekly) can lead to constipation. "There is also a concern that large amounts of calcium carbonate may cause acid rebound," says Dr. Giacona. "That's when excessive acid is produced several hours after a dose of calcium antacid, setting up a possible vicious circle of acid secretion, antacid, acid, antacid, and so forth."

In one study of 24 patients with chronic duodenal ulcers, taking four to eight grams of calcium carbonate induced excessive acid secretion 3 to 5.5 hours later, whereas two to four tablespoons of aluminum hydroxide of four to eight grams of sodium bicarbonate did not (*Handbook of Nonprescription Drugs,* American Pharmaceutical Association).

Nevertheless, adds Charles B. Clayman, M.D., of Northwestern University Medical School, in Chicago, "No one has shown that any of this has clinical bearing on the effectiveness of calcium antacids in the treatment of peptic ulcer."

Indeed, even the threat of kidney-stone formation or hypercalcemia (excessive calcium in the blood) has been overplayed, Dr. Giacona says. "Our bodies are designed to compensate for variations of calcium intake. Unless a person has kidney disease, where the mechanisms break down and you can't eliminate the excess amount, those problems are uncommon. In fact, if you are taking a calcium supplement, it very likely is calcium carbonate—the same ingredient as the antacid, just without the flavorings that the antacid product has."

Magnesium Hydroxide

Magnesium hydroxide (Philips Milk of Magnesia) has less neutralizing capability than the two previous antacids mentioned but is still
very effective. Magnesium is rarely used as the only ingredient in a
product, however, because of its well-known laxative effect. Most often
it is used in combination with aluminum-containing antacid to counteract the constipation that commonly occurs with those products.

Magnesium-containing antacids pose a different threat to people
with kidney disease, though. If excess magnesium can't be eliminated
from your body, it may accumulate in your blood, causing a condition
called hypermagnesemia. When that happens your blood pressure
drops, there's nausea, vomiting and ultimately, coma.

Aluminum Hydroxide

Aluminum hydroxide (AlternaGEL, Amphojel) is the weakest of the
acid neutralizers and is rarely used as the sole active ingredient. Most
often it is found in combination with magnesium products (Gelusil,
Maalox, Mylanta), with sodium bicarbonate (Rolaids), or with calcium
and magnesium (Tempo, Camalox).

Although constipation is the main side effect of aluminum-containing
antacids, it is not the one that causes the greatest concern. Doctors
used to think that aluminum passed through the body without being
absorbed into the bloodstream. Now research has shown that not only
is part of it absorbed but that some of it also binds with dietary
phosphate and calcium, dragging them out of the body and possibly
weakening the bones.

In one study, researchers decided to test the effects on phosphorus
and calcium metabolism using small doses of aluminum-containing
antacids. Seventeen men participated in the study and were given at
least two tablespoons of antacid three times a day for a maximum of 36
days. The doctors also kept a check of each volunteer's dietary calcium
and phosphorus intake. The researchers found that even with small
doses of aluminum-containing antacids, there was a significant increase
in the amount of calcium and phosphorus excreted from the body
(*American Journal of Clinical Nutrition,* July, 1982).

"Phosphorus depletion," says Herta Spencer, M.D., one of the researchers who conducted the study, "has been reported to stimulate bone resorption [loss], and this process would result in removal of both phosphorus and calcium from bone, thereby leading to an increase in urinary calcium. . . . The calcium loss induced by either increased bone resorption or decreased mineralization may eventually result in skeletal demineralization."

Indeed, says Dr. Spencer, "osteomalacia [adult rickets] has been reported in antacid-induced phosphorus depletion." What's more, this release of calcium from the bones can lead to or worsen osteoporosis, a bone-weakening disease.

On a more positive note, Dr. Spencer's study also showed that when calcium intake was approximately 800 milligrams per day (that's close to the Recommended Dietary Allowance—RDA) these antacids did *not* result in a significant increase in calcium excretion, indicating that a diet high in calcium may reduce or counteract the antacid-induced bone resorption observed during low calcium intake.

Doctors now know that some aluminum is absorbed *into* the body, as well, and that an accumulation of aluminum in the brain has been related to Alzheimer's disease, a brain disorder that accounts for about half of the cases of senility. "There is no proof, however, that aluminum causes the disease," Dr. Giacona cautions. "It may be that the disease itself has made those brain cells more permeable to aluminum."

Bursting Bubbles

You may have noticed that some products (Di-gel, Maalox Plus) offer an additional ingredient called simethicone, specifically designed to reduce gas bubbles. There's some question as to whether the claims are justified. The Food and Drug Administration says that simethicone is "safe and effective," but some doctors have their doubts. "The clinical data is scanty," says Dr. Giacona, "but there are some patients who swear by it. So, if it works for you, then use it."

There's no doubt, however, that antacids have made it easy to eliminate heartburn and acid indigestion. It's one thing to use them for an occasional attack of heartburn or indigestion and quite another to be popping tablets several times a day. "Any digestive symptoms that last more than two weeks should be checked out by a physician," advises Dr. Giacona, "since antacids may mask a more serious medical problem. For example, if your heartburn isn't immediately relieved with an antacid, the pain may be from angina, not indigestion—a symptom requiring prompt medical supervision."

For those with simple, occasional acid indigestion, a standard dose of any of the antacids will do the job, say the experts. Liquids work faster because there is more surface area exposed to the acid, but tablets are more convenient. Check the prices—and then pick the least expensive one with the ingredient you can tolerate best, and the taste and form (liquid or tablet) most pleasing to you.

It's best to take antacids on a full stomach. On an empty stomach, antacids work only from 20 to 40 minutes. Taken one hour after eating, however, they continue to neutralize acid for up to three hours. Also, antacids interact with certain antibiotics, heart medications and other drugs, so check with your doctor or pharmacist before taking them. And it's still best to try to eliminate the cause of your digestive problem rather than accepting antacid gobbling as a way of life.

Preventing Indigestion

Here are a few hints:

• Cut out caffeine-containing beverages. They increase acid production in the stomach.

• Avoid irritant foods, such as citrus juice, tomatoes and spicy foods.

• Avoid chocolate, alcohol, spearmint, peppermint and smoking. They lower esophageal sphincter pressure.

• Avoid fatty foods and large meals, which reduce gastric emptying.

• Wait at least three hours following a meal before going to bed.

• Raise the head of your bed six to eight inches to improve stomach emptying.

• Avoid stooping or exercises that compress your stomach.

• Lose weight if necessary.

CHAPTER 3

All about Antihistamines

There's something in the air—pollen. And for something that you can't even see, it can make a mighty nuisance of itself if it happens to pick on allergic you when it's ready to come in for a landing.

That heady, heavy, drippy, sneezy, itchy feeling is the classic sign of the seasonal condition known as hay fever, which makes its way into one out of ten sets of nostrils every fall. The symptoms are caused by the release of a body chemical called histamine, which is set off by the presence of pollen. And short of taking a cruise in the mid-Atlantic or holing up in a room with an air conditioner, hay fever's victims must face the consequences.

Its name is really a misnomer, for it has nothing to do with hay and rarely causes fever. But it has been known to spark some emotional heat in its victims when it comes to seeking some relief in a tablet.

Anyone who's ever had a brush with this late-summer nag knows that the over-the-counter counterattack to histamine comes from a chemical substance called antihistamine. Sounds simple enough, but it really isn't. There are literally hundreds of antihistamine drugs on the market. Finding a worthwhile one, to put it mildly, can be aggravating. And judging from the millions after millions of dollars spent each year on hay-fever medications, there are an awful lot of blind decisions taking place this very minute.

One way you might be tempted to cut down on the myriad of possibilities facing you on the drugstore shelf is to eliminate all the ones you can't pronounce. It most definitely would cut down your choices considerably. But, of course, it wouldn't be a very smart thing to do. For there's one very important thing to keep in mind: If relief from natural remedies is coming too slowly and you feel the faster route to relief is with antihistamines, make sure you choose your drug wisely. Some contain compounds to treat symptoms you may not have. You certainly don't need that. Then there is drowsiness, an almost certain side effect, although it can vary from product to product.

"For pure hay-fever sufferers, over-the-counter hay-fever medications can provide relief—the same relief you can get from a prescription drug," says Jeremy H. Thompson, M.D., of the department of pharmacology at UCLA. "The problem is that what works for some people won't necessarily work for others. So you have to try different types to find one that works." But it's only the antihistamine and not the other ingredients in a tablet that is stopping the action of histamine and doing the job against hay-fever symptoms.

It makes sense to stick with a simple antihistamine, and nothing more, when it comes to choosing a hay-fever aid. Unfortunately, once again it's not as simple as it may sound. Antihistamines come in five basic chemical types, which are subdivided into a variety of tongue-twisting names. And unless you're a chemist or a wizard at linguistics, reading the ingredients can leave you scratching your head.

Even if the label just contains one ingredient—one long ingredient—it can be confusing to the consumer. And that's where a second bit of sensible advice comes in.

Talk to a Pharmacist

"Never pick up a product without knowing what you're buying just because you heard it was good," says Stephen H. Paul, Ph.D., of Temple University School of Pharmacy. "Go to a drugstore where you know the pharmacist. Explain your symptoms to him—if you have a runny nose, if the liquid is dripping into your throat. He'll direct you to the product. With the hundreds of products on the market that fall into different categories, it only makes sense to seek help from a qualified professional."

Let's back up a bit. To best understand all the ramifications of antihistamine medications, it's necessary to know exactly how they work.

When pesky pollen comes in for its attack, it causes an allergic reaction in sensitive individuals which, in turn, triggers the release of histamine from the tissues. While histamine is available throughout the body, it's the area around the head, and most notably the nose, where all the action takes place. Tissue surfaces contain receptor sites that attract the histamine. When histamine hits, the classic reactions occur—redness, swelling, itching, runny nose and runny eyes. But if an antihistamine gets to the receptor site first, the histamine can't do its dirty work. Unfortunately, not all receptor sites are equal.

Receptor sites can also react differently at different times. You just may find that what works today won't necessarily work tomorrow. "A drug that you find works very well can gradually lose its effectiveness," says Dr. Thompson. "A tolerance develops. You'll find you'll have to switch to another product, which may or may not work at all. But the same goes for the drowsiness. Some people can build up a tolerance to this side effect."

Staying Alert

Serious side effects, he says, are rare in healthy teenagers and adults. But the drowsiness can cause calamitous results if used in combination with other sedation-inducing drugs, such as alcohol, tranquilizers and barbiturates.

"The important thing to remember is that the side effects of the drug are not necessarily dangerous," says Dr. Thompson. "It's not knowing what the side effects are that can be dangerous. You should never drink alcoholic beverages, drive a car or operate heavy machinery while taking antihistamines."

That was well established when a group of Australian students volunteered to measure the effects of antihistamines alone and in combination with a "social dose" of alcohol. A control group taking a placebo (harmless blank pill) was also used. Steadiness, reaction time, manual dexterity and perceptual speed were all affected by the combination of drug and alcohol. In fact, when it came to reaction time there was no difference between the alcohol users and the placebo users. But there was a noticeable slowdown in reaction time when the antihistamine was combined with the alcohol (*Medical Journal of Australia,*

April 22, 1978). The researchers warned that the combination "might represent a safety factor in the driving situation."

But there still remains the big question. Just what should you look for? As we said, antihistamines are divided into five chemical compounds, but only three are basic hay-fever medications: The alkylamines generally have the least sedative effect; the ethanolamines have the most sedative effect; and the ethylenediamines fall somewhere in the middle. All are available in a wide list of generic names and under many trade names. For example, one very popular antihistamine is chlorpheniramine maleate, a type of alkylamine. But, as pharmacologist Joe Graedon points out in his book *The People's Pharmacy* (St. Martin's Press), it is available in some 65 over-the-counter formulations, most of which contain a whole slew of other questionable ingredients, such as caffeine, aspirin, sleep inducers, decongestants and other drying agents. But what you want to do is find a product that contains the antihistamine alone. Again, ask your pharmacist for help.

Also, some brands contain a combination of two or three antihistamines. However, there is no evidence that these have an advantage over taking a single dose of one antihistamine in its full therapeutic amount.

And while hay fever can feel like a cold that just never goes away, you should never confuse the two conditions. There is a big difference between hay fever and a cold. Likewise, there is a big difference between what works for each and what doesn't.

"A cold is caused by a virus and hay fever is the result of a release of histamine and other substances," says Dr. Thompson. "Antihistamines block the activity of histamine but they have no action against the symptoms of a common cold."

Another thing to keep in mind about antihistamines is that they are best used to treat mild, seasonal suffering. More serious cases should receive a doctor's attention. Also antihistamines should never be taken without physician approval by people with high blood pressure, asthma, and glaucoma, men with urinary troubles and those who suffer from convulsions. And, it goes without saying that pregnant women and nursing mothers should avoid them altogether.

"For children and the elderly, the regular dosage should be cut back accordingly. Most packages contain this information. If not, consult your pharmacist," says Dr. Paul.

CHAPTER 4

All about Laxatives

L axatives are big business. Each year, in fact, we spend nearly $400 million on drugs that are supposed to bring us relief from that indelicate condition called constipation.

In a way, it's no wonder, because 41 million of us are plagued with constipation. And if you're one of the sufferers, you'll find more than 700 over-the-counter laxative products to choose from—a confusing situation, to say the least, especially since the active ingredients may vary from brand to brand.

Just because these drugs are available without a prescription, they're not necessarily safe. On the contrary, serious side effects are not uncommon with certain preparations.

The worst consequence is laxative abuse. That occurs when taking a laxative becomes so routine that it is virtually impossible to go without one. Year after year of laxative ingestion does not go unnoticed by your insides. According to Jacques Thiroloix, M.D., author of *Constipation: Its Causes and Cures* (St. Martin's Press), laxative sickness is almost inevitable when these products are taken for a long period of time. And the more toxic the laxative used, the sooner this condition appears.

"If laxatives are taken for a prolonged period, the chronic irritation will eventually alter the cells covering the internal wall of the colon [large intestine], exactly as if you'd sandpapered it every day," writes Dr. Thiroloix.

The results are devastating. The colon can no longer contract as it should, and normal intestinal muscle tone is shot. You're left with painful spasms—like colitis—where treatment leads, at best, to improvement but not cure. If you're smart you won't fall into that trap. There are safe ways to go about doing everything, and taking laxatives is no exception. Taken once in a while, laxatives are probably okay. But still, some are better than others. The best ones, according to the experts, help your own natural digestive processes along in the most harmless, gentle way. Here's how the major types of laxatives stack up.

• **Chemical stimulants** are the strongest and most-abused laxatives. Chemical names to look for are senna (Senokot, Fletcher's Castoria), phenolphthalein (Ex-Lax, Correctol, Feen-a-Mint), cascara and danthron (Dorbane), bisacodyl (Dulcolax) and castor oil. All of those chemicals work fast—usually in less than eight hours. Unfortunately, they may also produce painful cramps, diarrhea, dehydration and, when taken regularly, depletion of certain minerals from the body.

Doctors have advised against stimulant laxatives in general but have come down especially hard on the phenolphthalein ones. They're the most toxic of all the products that you could use for constipation, says Dr. Thiroloix. They act by irritating the colon wall. "The cells of the colon 'weep' under the assault, secreting a ropy, gluey liquid—mucus—which, mixing itself with the fecal mass, makes it more liquid."

The other chemical stimulants aren't much better. Bisacodyl can cause rectal burning. Senna and cascara are excreted in the breast milk of lactating women and can cause diarrhea in the infant. Danthron has been implicated in a case of hepatitis. And castor oil is potentially damaging to the lining of the small intestine.

• **Osmotic or saline (salt) laxatives** absorb and pull water into the feces for fast (in two to six hours) and often liquid relief. They are also quite potent—almost as potent as the chemical stimulants, in fact. The most common ones include magnesium hydroxide (milk of magnesia), magnesium sulfate (Epsom salts) and sodium sulfate.

Besides the unpleasant effect of liquid purge, these laxatives may pose a threat to patients with heart or kidney failure, due to excessive absorption of sodium or magnesium. What's more, the sodium laxatives can be harmful to those on a salt-restricted diet.

In this category, milk of magnesia is the mildest and could probably be tolerated if used infrequently.

Glycerin suppositories can also be classified here, too. They have no effect on the rest of the body, and they work in about 30 minutes. At worst, they can cause rectal irritation, but that's rare.

• **Lubricants** such as liquid paraffin and mineral oil at by coating the stool, allowing it easy passage.

Even though lubricants have been around for eons, doctors now feel that these agents should not be used in treating constipation. That's because, taken over a long period, mineral oil may deplete the body of all the fat-soluble vitamins (A, D, E, K). Besides, it can be messy, since it sometimes causes rectal leakage. It's even been suspected of causing an increased risk of gastrointestinal malignancies.

• **Stool softeners** are like detergents. They promote the mixture of water and fatty substances, which then penetrate the stool and soften it. The chemical involved is called DDS—dioctyl sodium sulfosuccinate (Colace). Although DDS does not interfere with the absorption of nutrients from the intestinal tract, it has been reported to enhance the absorption of mineral oil and should never be used along with it. About the only time that stool softeners are really useful is after a heart attack or rectal surgery, when straining should be avoided.

• **Bulk-forming agents** include psyllium preparations (Metamucil, Effersyllium, Konsyl), polycarbophil (Mitrolan) and plantago (Siblin). They work by absorbing water and expanding. The added bulk stimulates contractions, while the absorbed water softens and fluffs up stools, making them easier to pass. These agents take a while to work—from one to three days. Their main function is to *prevent* rather than treat constipation.

Until recently, several of these products have been high in sodium, but manufacturers have since cut it back considerably. However, many still contain much sugar. What's more, bulk formers must be taken with at least eight ounces of water (or other fluid) to prevent a possible blockage of the gastrointestinal tract. Still, bulking agents are about the safest laxatives you can take, probably because they encourage your own system to do the work.

Eat plenty of unrefined bran, vegetable and fruit fibers and whole grains—nature's bulk-forming agents—and you'll probably have no need for commercial bulk-forming products or other laxatives.

CHAPTER 5

Diet Pills: The Facts, the Lies, the Surprises

"**K**iss the fat goodbye! Explosive new fat burn-off system with once-a-day pill is so surefire it's the ultimate weapon against fat! Now you can quickly drop 10, 20, 50 pounds or more! Best of all, your weight loss is achieved without torturous starvation, agonizing exercise or dangerous drugs! You can have exciting meal after meal, delicious snack after snack, while at the same time slashing your calorie intake!"

Seems too good to be true, doesn't it?

So to entice you further, each ad is accompanied by a picture of a gorgeous, thin, bikini-clad model or a tight-muscled man. You sigh wistfully, dreaming of someday looking just like that.

Then your common sense snaps you back to reality, and you instinctively know that the model's closest encounter with fat was probably the dictionary. Besides, losing weight can't be all *that* easy or no one in the world would be fat.

Still, when you're overweight, desperate and hungry, part of you clings to the possibility that maybe there's some truth to the hype. After all, some of the ads do say, "doctor tested and approved by the U.S. government." They claim to have "scientific proof" that you can "shed fat even if you eat more." And they insist that the pills are "safe, gentle and effective." They couldn't print that if it weren't true, could they? Of course not. But first they have to be caught. Meanwhile, the facts are mixed in with the fiction, and it's up to you to sort out one from the other.

Believe it or not, a few of the claims made in those ads are actually true (we'll let you know which ones). But most of them are outright lies and a blatant attempt at consumer fraud.

So, don't get your hopes up. By taking those pills, you've got much more to lose then your fat. We're talking about putting a crimp in your pocketbook and, more important, in your health.

A Drug That Tricks Your Brain

Over-the-counter (OTC) reducing aids, which include candy, gum, tablets, time-release capsules and drops, are meant to curb your appetite— and that's all! Most often they do that with a drug called phenylpro-panolamine (PPA), a laboratory-produced chemical similar to epineph-rine (adrenaline), a hormone naturally produced by the adrenal glands.

When you take PPA, it affects the hypothalamus, a portion of the brain that regulates the appestat (appetite control center). Apparently PPA persuades your appestat that you're not hungry, so you eat less and hence lose weight.

Some of the pills contain only PPA. Others may be laced with caffeine (as much as 200 milligrams—the equivalent of two cups of coffee) or diuretics. The caffeine acts as a stimulant to relieve the fatigue often associated with reducing diets. Meanwhile, the diuretic gives you the impression of rapid weight loss when, if fact, it's only water that's come off, not fat.

If you've bought a chewing gum or candy diet aid, it most likely contains benzocaine, a mild topical anesthetic like that used in throat lozenges. In fact, it works the same way. It numbs the taste buds on your tongue, so food won't taste as good, and, theoretically, you'll eat less.

So much for the fact. "The rest is pure fiction," says James Ramey, M.D., assistant clinical professor of medicine at George Washington University Medical School in Washington, D.C., and a specialist in endocrinology and metabolism. "Those over-the-counter diet pills absolutely will not do the things those ads say. There is no way you can eat more and lose weight, for example. Those claims are all nonsense."

Even the ability of PPA to suppress appetite is exaggerated. "It will curb it somewhat," says Dr. Ramey "but not much and not for very long, either."

Effects Don't Last Long

"Your body can even build up a tolerance to phenylpropanolamine. Besides, the effects are short-lived and minimal. And there's always the possibility of a psychological dependence on the drug, too."

Besides that, diet pills are expensive. It seems the more outrageous the claims in the advertisements, the higher the price of the product. It's still PPA, but the cost can be anywhere from two to five times more for some pills than others.

And while the ads claim you can still eat all you want, once the pills arrive you'll notice that the package includes recommendations for a highly restricted, low-calorie diet. In other words, you still have to cut calories to lose weight. Only that's not what the original ad said. You are, in fact, paying a very high price (as much as $9 for a 10-day supply of pills) and at best getting an ordinary diet plan, the sort available in weekly magazines.

With those kinds of prices, over-the-counter diets aids have become big business. According to one estimate, about $110 million a year is spent on such products. And that's expected to increase in the future.

And no wonder. With about 50 million overweight people in the United States, there's a never-ending supply of possible consumers.

So drug companies continue to exploit the American passion to be thin. And they practically have the endorsement of the Food and Drug Administration (FDA), to boot.

In May, 1979, a panel of physicians and scientists (one of 17 established by the FDA to review the safety and effectiveness of all over-the-counter drugs) concluded that PPA and benzocaine may help people lose weight safely.

The FDA panel based its determination of the drugs' effectiveness for weight control on studies that are not described, and whose authors are not identified. The panel found those studies "defective in one or more important facets" but concluded, nevertheless, that the unidentified, defective studies, taken all together, established the effectiveness of the drugs (*Medical Letter,* August 10, 1979).

Label Claims Forbidden

Advertisers jumped on that information, even though the FDA still hasn't completed its evaluation of the panel's report. In fact, the panel itself states flatly that labels of OTC weight-control drugs should not carry undocumented or misleading claims like "contains one of the most powerful diet aids available without prescription," "trims pounds and inches without crash diets or strenuous exercise," "the modern aid to appetite control" or "removes excess body weight" (*FDA Consumer,* October, 1979).

Since the pills are only for curbing or controlling appetite, that is precisely the *only* claim the advertisers are allowed to make—legally, that is.

So why have those rules been all but ignored? "We on the staff are very concerned about it," says Joel Brewer of the Federal Trade Commission (FTC). "In fact we've already gone after one advertiser who made false weight-loss claims. In 1977 the FTC prohibited marketers of 'X-11' diet aid from stating that their pill has a unique ingredient allowing people to lose weight without eating less.

"So the precedent has been set," says Brewer, "and that helps when it comes to prosecuting other offenders." Still, the FTC could not say whether other suits are pending in that area, even though it seems clear that the advertisers are in violation of the truth-in-advertising laws.

Actually, they're as much in violation for what they *don't* print as for what they do. The government requires a warning stating the possible hazard of using PPA when other conditions exist or when other drugs are being taken. And with good reason, too.

It's all too easy to overdose on PPA without even knowing it. That's because PPA is the main ingredient used in nasal decongestants like Contac, Alka Seltzer Plus cold medicine, Vicks Day Care, Comtrex and Sinarest.

At this writing the FDA says that 75 milligrams of PPA is the maximum dose allowed for diet pills in any 24-hour period. But if you have a cold or a sinus condition and are taking one of the medications mentioned above, you could be getting as much as 267 milligrams of PPA in one day!

It's true that the dosages are spread out over a 24-hour period— but not as much as you might like to believe. "Timed-release capsules, in theory, are supposed to spread out their doses over a period of 12 hours," says Solomon Snyder, M.D., a professor of psychiatry and pharmacology at John Hopkins University School of Medicine in Baltimore. "But they really don't. You reach the peak of the dose in the bloodstream fairly soon after taking the pill. After that it slowly declines. I worry about what that could do to blood pressure."

Can Raise Blood Pressure

Lots, apparently. A recent study done at the University of Melbourne in Australia showed just how serious the effects could be. Researchers divided 72 healthy young medical students with normal blood pressure into two groups. One group (37) took Trimolets (a diet pill containing 85 milligrams of PPA per capsule), while the other group (35) was given a placebo (a harmless blank pill).

Blood pressure reached a peak between 1½ and 3 hours after the Trimolets were given. In 12 out of the 37 (33 percent), diastolic blood pressure rose to a dangerously high level. Only one of the 35 taking the placebo had that effect. Three of the subjects taking the Trimolets actually required treatment for their high blood pressure.

"The current study demonstrated that in a large group of young normotensive [normal-blood-pressure] adults, important and sometimes dangerous rises in blood pressure may occur after ingestion of a single capsule of phenylpropanolamine-containing preparation.

"Furthermore," say the researchers, "a report of cerebral hemorrhage after ingestion of Trimolets confirms that these adverse effects may be life threatening" (*Lancet,* January 12, 1980).

Because of the alarming blood pressure effects, reseachers discontinued the study of Trimolets and substituted a decongestant that contains a smaller dose of PPA (50 milligrams). It, too, was found likely to induce high blood pressure, especially if more than one capsule is taken.

But it wasn't just high blood pressure that the medical students experienced. Nearly half taking the Trimolets reported symptoms of dizziness, headache, chest tightness, rash, nausea or palpitations. The occurrence of symptoms corresponded closely with the increase in blood pressure in each person tested.

Psychotic Episodes

In fact, because of the results of the Australian study, the FDA decided to keep the maximum dose at 75 milligrams instead of following the recommendation of the advisory panel to raise the maximum to 150 milligrams per day.

And it's a good thing they did, too. Because high doses of PPA can cause more than elevated blood pressure. The drug can literally drive you crazy.

That's what Charles B. Schaffer, M.D., reports. There have been cases of psychotic episodes in several patients following use of PPA as a decongestant and in a woman taking OTC diet pills. Dr. Schaffer, a psychiatrist affiliated with the University of California, Davis, School of Medicine, says the woman displayed startling changes in behavior: She made bizarre and paranoid statements and believed people were going to harm her. Her thoughts were disorganized, and her judgment was impaired.

"The acute psychotic episode experienced by this patient," says Dr. Schaffer, "was most likely related to the ingestion of more than the recommended amount of [the drugs]. Her psychiatric symptoms began shortly after her indiscreet self-medication, and resolved quickly without treatment after these agents were discontinued" (*American Journal of Psychiatry,* October, 1980).

"The wide use of phenylpropanolamine as a decongestant for colds, hay fever and sinusitis, plus its increasing use as an oral over-the-counter anorexic [appetite-suppressing] agent," concludes Dr. Schaffer, "indicates a need to increase our awareness of its possible serious psychiatric side effects, including psychotic reactions."

In addition, one report implicates PPA as a possible cause of kidney failure in a patient who also took two or three tablets of aspirin and acetaminophen, an aspirin substitute (*Lancet,* July 7, 1979).

In another, the PPA in one capsule of a cold remedy was thought to contribute to a fatal heart attack in a patient taking thioridazine, an antidepressant (*Canadian Medical Association Journal,* October 7, 1978).

And a third states that high blood pressure crises can occur when PPA is used at the same time as antidepressant drugs containing monoamine oxidase (MAO) inhibitors (*Medical Letter,* March 10, 1979).

More recently, Albert J. Dietz, Jr., M.D., Ph.D., reports that seven women experienced symptoms ranging from tremor and restlessness to agitation and hallucinations after taking just one PPA tablet. Dr. Dietz, from the department of internal medicine at the University of

North Dakota School of Medicine in Fargo, says, "Physicians should be alerted to the possible side effects from ingesting preparations containing phenylpropanolamine. Warnings on products containing PPA should include the serious [central nervous system] effects of the agent" (*Journal of the American Medical Association,* February 13, 1981).

It's easy to see why diet pills should not be taken by people with high blood pressure, depression or kidney and heart disease. But they're also a no-no for those with diabetes or thyroid disease, says the FDA. And a warning stating just that should be clearly printed on the label and should appear in the advertisements for those products— especially since a substantial number of overweight individuals suffer from one or more of those conditions. Yet, about half the ads in the magazines we examined fail to say anything at all about such possible dangers.

And even when they do, the print is so small it's virtually impossible to read.

"Indeed, the risks of these anorexic agents as diet aids may outweigh their benefits," says Dr. Schaffer, "because there is no reliable evidence that PPA can help obese patients achieve long-term weight reduction."

Virgil Jennings, D.O., a specialist in preventive medicine and weight loss from Fort Worth, Texas, agrees. "Without changing your diet and understanding nutrition, the weight loss will not be permanent," he says.

"Besides," says Dr. Ramey, "those pills do not curb desire. So if your appetite for food is unrelated to hunger, as it is in many obese people, they will not have an appetite-suppressing effect at all. "And even if they do suppress your appetite, it will not be by much or for long. And you're taking a real chance of having adverse effects."

Unfortunately, there is no "magic bullet" to help you lose weight permanently. But there are those who will take your money for a bottle of lies and only a slim chance of losing a few pounds.

CHAPTER 6

Seven Signs of a Good Doctor

Can you tell a good doctor from a bad one? If your town had only two physicians, could you pick the better one? Making such distinctions could be a lifesaving act, yet few of us know how to go about it.

Some people may make a serious effort, only to use the wrong yardsticks to measure a doctor's worth. As a case in point, try sizing up this professional healer. Doctor X got his* M.D. from an Ivy League medical school, has a wallful of framed certificates from medical examining boards and has staff privileges at three medical centers. The local medical society gives out his name to people seeking a family physician.

So is he likely to be a good medical man? Don't bet your life on it. Fact is, it's impossible to answer the question based on the credentials listed. Despite what some consumer-advocacy groups suggest, such information doesn't tell you a thing about the quality of care you can expect from a physician.

"Knowing where a doctor got his medical education is no help," says George D. LeMaitre, M.D., distinguished senior surgeon at Bon

---

*The authors are aware that your doctor may be man or a woman. We have used masculine pronouns for the sake of simplicity.

Secours Hospital, near Boston. "All medical schools in this country are fully accredited and offer their students a high-quality education. But even the finest training in the world won't guarantee that a physician will be responsible and conscientious. Board certification is a minimum standard of excellence, nothing more. The problem is that *most* graduate physicians of recent years have their boards, just as almost all doctors have hospital privileges. And calling the local medical society for recommendations gets you nowhere. Medical societies aren't referral agencies. They can give you a list of physicians in your area, but they can't tell you which ones are good and which bad."

Dr. LeMaitre, author of *How to Choose a Good Doctor* (Andover), points out that the popular credentials-checking approach rests on the shaky premise that a piece of paper, such as a diploma or a board certificate, proves that a doctor is sterling. "But no amount of documentation with medical credentials guarantees professional excellence," he says. "Good doctors are good because of certain characteristics they have—most of which can't be measured by quantitative means."

A lot of patients and medical professionals concur. And there seems to be plenty of agreement on what some of those characteristics are. The following seven are at the top of the list.

1. Good Doctors Avoid Overdoctoring

Overdoctoring happens when your physician orders a battery of tests on you though one or two would do. Or hospitalizes you for x-rays and blood work though you could get the same tests as an outpatient. Or is quick to reach for the prescription pad without considering non-drug remedies.

"Doctors are taught to rely heavily on tests and drugs," says Tom Ferguson, M.D., editor of *Medical Self-Care* magazine. "Even though it might be more effective in certain cases for a doctor to spend 45 minutes personally exploring a patient's complaints and symptoms, many physicians would opt to spend only 10 minutes doing that and then order up a lot of tests or medication. They hope that such overdoctoring makes up for time not spent in the examining room."

Critics of the medical profession point out that overdoctoring can be very profitable for physicians. Not to mention fascinating. To some doctors, sophisticated tests and fancy medications have enormous appeal. A good doctor, however, finds ways to wield the technology with proper restraint.

2. Good Doctors Avoid Underdoctoring

This is the sin of omission—failure to follow up on your prescribed treatment, to attend to every significant detail of your illness, to work hard at preventing and curing disease.

"Underdoctoring," says Dr. LeMaitre, "exists when your doctor removes a wart from your arm (for $40) because you requested it and fails to remove that pack of cigarettes from your pocket or at least talk it over with you. Underdoctoring occurs when your doctor observes that your blood pressure has increased but fails to note that your waistline has, too. The old-time doctor got angry with his patient for pushing too hard or drinking too much. The modern physician gets angry with the lab for being late with your blood test report."

Underdoctoring is usually not a failure of a physician's intellect but of his attitude, says Dr. LeMaitre. "Observe the little things he does, not the big words he uses. The tests he orders are not half as important as your test of how much he cares about you. Underdoctoring exists when diseases are discovered and treated in a vacuum, disconnected from the patient and unrelated to his loved ones."

3. Good Doctors Know the Value of Time

They don't make you cool your heels in their waiting room for an hour or more at each visit, and they don't hustle you through an examination as though you were a gizmo on an assembly line.

Some people have come up against the long wait in the doctor's office so often that they think of it as a natural part of doctoring. But most patients resent those lengthy delays, and some outspoken physicians have declared them bad medicine. After all, they contend, patients have schedules, too.

Of course, if a doctor suddenly has an accident victim on his hands or discovers that a patient has a bleeding ulcer or is threatened by a heart attack, that's a different story. "Naturally these emergencies require extra time and effort on the part of the physician and his office staff," says Lewis Miller, former editor of *Medical Economics* and author of *The Life You Save* (Berkley). "They cannot be anticipated, and most people are understanding about delays of this nature."

But the *routine* lengthy delay—anything over 30 minutes, some experts say—should raise both your eyebrows. Chances are it means the doctor has overbooked his patients. Overbooking may raise his income, but it's not likely to help him give you better care.

A growing number of physicians agree: Good doctoring takes time—time to formulate an accurate diagnosis, time to explain to the patient what the problem is and what's to be done about it.

So if you're in and out of your doctor's office in nothing flat, maybe you should stay away from his revolving door. And if he can't give you his undivided attention once he's granted you the time, maybe you should find a doctor who can. Miller warns you to be on the lookout for "the doctor who has four or five patients in different treatment rooms, and runs back and forth from one to another instead of dealing fully with one patient before going to the next (alternating between *two* patients is often an efficient use of time) . . . the doctor whose nurse feels free to open the door and interrupt while he is examining or talking with the patient . . . the doctor who accepts nonemergency telephone calls while in the middle of examining or treating a patient."

4. Good Doctors Care about Your Diet

Does your doctor ever ask you what you eat? Does he try to assess your vitamin intake? Evidence demonstrating the powerful impact of nutrition on health has been piling up for decades. Yet many physicians, perhaps because of the dearth of nutritional training in medical schools, act as if nutrition was none of their business. Most of the doctors interviewed in a recent study, for example, said that they didn't know whether their patients used vitamin supplements and didn't think it was their responsibility to find out. Good doctors do find out, though, and they're just as eager to examine your diet as to check your blood pressure.

"Nutrition is such a major factor in a patient's health that it cannot be overestimated," says Arthur C. Hochberg, Ph.D., a nutritional psychologist at the Center of Preventive Medicine and Dentistry, in Bala Cynwyd, Pennsylvania. "It is absolutely essential that each doctor see the connection that nutrition has to health. I have had many patients who have been helped just by changing their nutrition around."

5. Good Doctors Are Good Teachers

"The word 'doctor' means teacher," says Dr. LeMaitre, "and it is the doctor's responsibility to teach his patients the art of healthy living. Those patients who are in excellent health must be taught how to preserve it. Those who have an ailment, whether acute or chronic, must be taught how to restore and maintain their health in the best possible state under the circumstances."

Dr. LeMaitre asserts that the single most important question you must ask yourself after visiting your doctor is this: How well do I understand my body, its illnesses, the drugs I'm to take, the tests I'm to have, and the regimen I must follow to keep my health or restore it? If you haven't the slightest idea, your doctor is not a teacher. School is out.

Polling surveys indicate that most Americans would prefer to get advice on diet, exercise and smoking from physicians but usually walk out of the doctor's office without it. A physician who teaches is golden.

6. Good Doctors Are Good Listeners

"Keep your mouth shut the first four or five minutes of the interview." That's the advice on talking with patients that one doctor offers his fellow physicians. He tenders these words to the wise because they're

33

obviously needed. Studies confirm what patients have grumbled about for years: Some doctors just don't know how to lend an ear. They interrupt, cut the conversation short, split their attention between you and the patient down the hall, and keep a sharp eye on the clock, ready to bolt when your time is up. Their inattention isn't simply a defense against those few patients who ramble on about trivia and waste a doctor's time. It's a habit of screening out cues from every patient who walks into the office.

"When patients visit a doctor, they may not want to state the obvious reason for illness," says Siegfried J. Kra, M.D., author of *Examine Your Doctor* (Tichnor and Fields). "A good doctor tries to pinpoint those reasons. He tries, for example, to make sure that that pain in the stomach is not a symptom of depression. Uncovering the real cause of illness means listening—and listening intently—to what the patient has to say."

7. Good Doctors Are Honest

They don't lie to themselves and they don't lie to you. If they're uncertain about your illness, if they don't have the answers, they don't pretend to be gods. They admit their limitations.

"Doctors have to be honest about what they know and don't know," says Dr. Kra. "They should be secure enough to say, 'I don't know. Let's get a second opinion.'"

They also should care enough about you to level with you about your illness. For it's only when you get a true picture of your condition that you can mobilize all your inner resources to get well. "When patients are kept in the dark about their illness, they can become passive," Dr. Hochberg says. "And it's difficult for passive patients to get well. But when a doctor gives them all the facts, they can free up their natural resistance to illness and fight it with clear determination."

CHAPTER 7

How to Be a Good Patient

"**V**ery often," reports Fred Scialabba, M.D., a New Jersey neurosurgeon, "I'll walk into my office and a patient will start machine-gunning me with complaints. So the times when a patient says, 'Hello, how're ya doin' Doc?' I feel really good."

As Dr. Scialabba says, "It's just a simple thing, but it makes the whole situation more relaxed." And it lets the physician feel like a person, not just a health provider.

What's the difference? Maybe a whole new way of looking at doctor-patient relationships.

Most of us already realize that medical care is not something to approach passively. We have to be informed, selective and questioning. We're aware of the possibility of unnecessary procedures. We know that even the best medications may produce terrible side effects. So we've learned to treat the physician like a consultant—not a boss—and demand that health care satisfy *our* needs, not those of the physician.

And that's smart. Except when we find ourselves treating the health professional like a health machine. When doctors start voicing the same complaints we patients used to spout—things like "You're treating me like an object" and "You don't listen"—then the quality of care we experience could well be headed down, not up.

To complete the health-care partnership, say experts in human communication, you must realize one inescapable fact: Doctors are people, too.

"Just like with anybody else, if you make a connection with a physician, you'll probably get along better," observes New York psychoanalyst Rema Greenberg. She suggests doing this with short, personal conversation, such as asking about the doctor's family. Maryellyn Duane, Ph.D., a New York psychologist/psychoanalyst, agrees. She says, "You should treat your physician the same way you would treat anybody socially: Be open, friendly and take an interest in the doctor as a person. Notice what the doctor's hobbies might be," she adds. "Is there fishing paraphernalia or a family snapshot around? Ask about it."

But both Dr. Duane and Rema Greenberg warn against seeing the rules of polite conversation as tricks to get the physician to react well to you. Simply be yourself and keep in mind that the doctor is just like you, but with a different area of expertise.

And keep in mind that, like you, physicians react to the way they are treated. Dr. Scialabba, for instance, finds it difficult to be positive with some of his more negative patients. "One time I greeted a patient as she came into the waiting room," he related. "I asked her how she was feeling—just being friendly, you know? And she answered, 'Terrible, terrible. Nothing you could help me with.' And that was in the waiting room. I was shot down before I even got a crack at her and that put me on the defensive with her," he remembers.

Of course, you're not always the cause of a physician's rude or abrupt manner. Consider the doctor who has spent an entire day seeing patients without making any headway. That's got to be pretty frustrating. So, if you're the 5:30 P.M. patient, a little sensitivity might loosen things up.

Susan Day, M.D., a general internist at the Hospital of the University of Pennsylvania, agrees. "When I'm really backed up and behind schedule, I always like it if a patient who's been waiting a long time acknowledges that I must be having a busy day instead of getting angry at me." She adds that, of course, it's not fair to *expect* a patient to do that. And Dr. Day is right—you don't *have* to treat the doctor like a person, but why not do it anyway? Most likely, it'll improve your relationship.

Of course, you don't want to be *too* nice; the passive or namby-pamby patient relates just as poorly as the abrasive patient. You've got to know certain things about a physician and you may need services that verge on being impositions. Still, there are friendly ways to ask for something. You might need a few forms filled out, for instance, or maybe a lot of forms. Really a lot. One New Jersey surgeon reports that whenever his Greek patients have an appointment, they come bearing gifts—cheesecake, cookies, sometimes tomatoes. And always reams of official rigamarole for him to sort out. "I know they bring the presents to get me to do them a favor," he says, "but I don't mind because I like getting presents. It puts me in a good mood." Maybe his patients' old-world generosity is going a bit far, but the premise—that doctors like to be treated kindly, too—might be worth keeping in mind.

It Pays to Be Pleasant

Even when you're well within your rights, the outcome is usually better if you're pleasant. If you don't like the way a doctor is treating you, suggests Stanley E. Sagov, M.D., author of *The Active Patient's Guide to Better Medical Care* (David McKay and Co.), assistant professor of family and community medicine at the University of Massachusetts, say something like, "Without meaning to offend you doctor, I would prefer it if you wouldn't do that."

You should always check into a potential doctor's credentials but Dr. Day warns that, "Asking someone how long they've been out of medical school isn't too healthy to the doctor-patient relationship."

Steven Schroeder, M.D., professor of medicine and chief of the division of general internal medicine at the University of California in San Francisco, is all for getting what you need from your doctor but has some ideas as to how such goals ought to be achieved. "I think it is true that the more demanding patients are, if they're nice about it, the more they are liable to get back," he says. "I have no problem with patients asking me questions about my own training or a treatment if it can be done nicely, with phrases like, 'Doc, I realize you're competent, but just to help me, could you review for me where you trained,' or 'Doctor, I don't mean to drag this interview out, but could you explain to me exactly what I need to take this medication and what the side effects could be.' Simple rules of tact and diplomacy work for everyone— family, friends and doctors alike."

Another big fan of tact is Emily Mumford, Ph.D., chief of the division of health utilization and policy research at the New York State Psychiatric Institute and professor of clinical social sciences at Columbia University. She advises, "Patients should realize doctors do have feelings. Most physicians have a sense of professionalism and of being right." So if you need or want a second opinion, you could soften the message by saying something like, "For my own peace of mind, I'd like to get a second opinion," or "My insurance coverage requires me to get a second opinion."

Act Naturally

Of course, if you really *don't* trust a physician, don't pretend you do. Honesty is what it all comes down to—honesty with the doctor and honesty with yourself. Playing manipulative games just isn't necessary. Mom told you before your first date to be yourself, and psychologists today say she was right. Acting naturally does pay off. "All people feel somewhat apprehensive about talking with doctors," observes Virginia Eman Wheeless, Ph.D., assistant professor of speech communication at Texas Tech University. "So it's hard to be yourself."

Concentrating on positive thoughts will help you relax and act naturally, says Dr. Duane. Some examples of positive thoughts are, "I'm in good hands," and "This is a pleasant experience."

And when you start to reap the benefits of an easy communication between you and your physician, it really will be a pleasant experience. "The payoff," says Dr. Wheeless, "is that you find out about your body and health care, and you learn more about how to take care of yourself." And once you and your doctor develop the habit of speaking openly with each other, the added knowledge you receive may not be just in response to your questions. Imagine going to the doctor for one problem and having him or her notice and offer advice on something you felt was too trivial to bring up. Now that's thorough medical care.

Dr. Wheeless also speculates that better communication could prove advantageous in terms of saving money. "For example," she says, "if you ask your doctor, 'Is it necessary for me to have an appointment with you every six months,' the answer could be 'No, just come once a year.'" Similarly, a doctor who communicates well with you might be inclined to suggest you change your own bandages or follow your child's illness on your own, thus saving costly medical bills.

CHAPTER 8

A Who's Who of Health Specialists

Remember when going to the doctor meant a short trip down the road to the neighborhood G.P.? You entrusted your health to this all-around practitioner, from the top of your head to the bottoms of your feet. After all, here was the supreme healer, the M.D.

Today, things aren't so simple and clear-cut. Medical specialties and alternative therapies abound. Some are old and some are new, but all have become more visible in today's consumer-oriented society. The name of the game is choice, and people have begun to shop around for the kind of health practitioner that will best fill their needs, whether it's an M.D., D.O. or D.C.

Still, unless you have a brother in the profession, it can be confusing. Is a D.D.S. the same as a D.M.D.? Can an osteopath do surgery? How is an optician different from an optometrist? What are naturopathic, homeopathic and orthomolecular medicine?

To sort it all out, we've put together a guide to the old and new specialties that have caused the most confusion and misunderstanding. Never again will you go to an *endodontist* for a hemorrhoid problem.

Medical Doctor (M.D.), Osteopathic Doctor (D.O.) and Chiropractic Doctor (D.C.)

Of course we all know what makes an M.D. Four years of college, three to five years of medical school and then a residency program for three or more years in one of many possible specialties that cover every inch of your body. What you may not realize is that D.O.'s are basically the same as M.D.'s—with one exception, manipulation (a form of manual pressure applied to joints, bones and muscles).

"M.D.'s and D.O.'s are the only practitioners who are legally called physicians," says Al Boeck, Ph.D., communications director of the American Osteopathic Association, in Chicago. "Both are *complete* physicians, too, meaning that they have received the same basic medical training and are licensed to treat the whole body, do surgery and prescribe drugs. The difference is that osteopathic physicians receive additional training in palpation and manipulative procedures, which they use along with the other more traditional forms of diagnosis and treatment.

"Actually some M.D.'s are now using manipulation in their practices, too. Only they call it biomechanics," says Dr. Boeck. "But it's really the same thing."

Chiropractors do manipulation, too. In fact, it's their stock-in-trade. But that's where the similarity to osteopaths ends. Although they study for four years at a special chiropractic college (after a minimum of two years at an undergraduate college), they are not licensed to do surgery or prescribe drugs, as D.O.'s and M.D.'s are.

Chiropractic doctors believe that spinal-nerve pressure or irritation can cause a disturbance of delicate body functions resulting in an increased susceptibility to disease. With the use of spinal adjustments (manipulation), a chiropractic doctor seeks to alleviate the irritation to the spinal nerves, thus curing the illness without drugs or surgery.

While chiropractors use other drugless therapies, such as heat, cold, water, massage, exercise and dietary management, spinal manipulation is still the dominant therapy for all ailments.

Podiatrist (D.P.M.) and Chiropodist

Actually these two names refer to the same specialty—diseases of the foot. "Up until 1958 we were known as chiropodists," says Louis G. Buttell, a director of public affairs for the American Podiatry Association, in Washington, D.C. "But chiropody actually means hands and feet. Since these specialists only treat feet, podiatry is a more accurate term."

That's not all that's changed over the years. "Seventy or 80 years ago you could become a podiatrist simply by completing a six-month course after high school. Today our students go through four years at a podiatric medical school and 90 to 95 percent have a bachelor of science (B.S.) degree before entering. After graduating, many go on to take a three-year hospital-based residency in podiatric surgery.

Podiatrists practicing today can do anything an M.D. can do except amputate," continues Buttell. "They handle breaks, sprains, artificial ankles, infections. In the last ten years sports injuries have become a big part of our practice, too. And many problems with the back and lower legs are often traceable to foot irregularities."

Optometrist, Optician and Ophthalmologist

If you are having a problem with your eyes, how do you know which of these people to see? "Both the optometrist and the ophthalmologist do complete eye-health examinations," says Charlotte Rancilio, news director of the American Optometric Association, in St. Louis, Missouri. "The difference comes not in the exam, but in the treatment. Since an ophthalmologist is an M.D. who specializes in diseases of the eye, he can perform surgery and treat all eye disorders or diseases. An optometrist cannot do all those things. His training, which includes four years at a school of optometry (with at least two or three years of undergraduate college), enables him to prescribe corrective lenses and other optical aids. He is also trained to diagnose certain diseases but he refers patients to an ophthalmologist for treatment.

"For example, glaucoma can be detected by an optometrist," Ms. Rancilio explained to us, "but the M.D. would be the one to treat it. On the other hand, the optometrist is trained to do vision therapy (eye exercises) and to help people with depth perception and eye tracking skills.

"An optician is basically the person who fills the lens prescriptions written by an optometrist or ophthalmologist. He cannot diagnose or treat eye diseases. The training may be on the job or include several years at a junior college. In some states opticians are allowed to fit contact lenses, but they can't prescribe them. That's the job of an optometrist or ophthalmologist."

41

Physician's Assistant (P.A.) and Nurse Practitioner (N.P.)

Neither of these health practitioners are doctors, but in many ways they do the work of physicians while under their supervision. It's been estimated that P.A.'s and N.P.'s can handle 70 to 80 percent of an M.D.'s practice. That's because most visits to a doctor's office involve minor but troublesome ailments such as colds, coughs, sore throats and earaches. Both N.P.'s and P.A.'s can also do case histories, diagnose and in some cases write prescriptions. And of course they know when to bring in the M.D. for problems they can't handle.

The differences between the two center mainly around their training. "Most people who come into the P.A. training program have had some medical background," says Peter Rosenstein, executive director of the American Academy of Physician's Assistants, in Arlington, Virginia. "They've worked in hospitals or in laboratories and they know they like that type of involvement. About 70 percent come into the program with a B.S. degree, but it's not an absolute necessity. The two-year P.A. course involves both book work and clinical experience with doctors. Right now there are about 15,000 P.A.'s working in the United States."

"Nurse practitioners are always nurses first," says Donna Diers, dean of the school of nursing at Yale University, in New Haven, Connecticut. "All have an R.N. and some have a B.S. degree. All have at least an additional 12 months' training in order to practice as an N.P."

Holistic, Homeopathic, Naturopathic and Orthomolecular Doctors

Here's where things start to get confusing. That's because some of these specialists are M.D.'s and some are not. And that's okay. It's just that it's important to know what you're getting. For instance, if someone says he's a holistic health practitioner, would you assume he's an M.D.? How about a homeopath or naturopath?

According to the Association for Holistic Health, in San Diego, California, "Applying the term holistic to the concept of health and fitness means that achieving and maintaining good health involves much more than just taking care of all the various components that make up the physical body. The individual is more than just the sum of the individual parts, and is the integration of the physical, the mental and the spiritual, united to form a unique being."

Holistic health practitioners stress prevention and help the patient develop healthy life patterns and attitudes. This approach is taken by many M.D.'s, but also by D.O.'s, chiropractors, nurses and others.

Homeopathic doctors, on the other hand, are *always* M.D.'s. Homeopathy is a formal branch of medicine, just as surgery is. Doctors who are homeopaths believe that you should treat an illness with something that produces an effect similar to the original suffering—"like heals like." The specially prepared substances used as remedies in homeopathy contain herbs, minerals or animal products (such as bee venom). These drugs are diluted so that only a minuscule amount actually enters a patient's body. With these products, homeopathic doctors treat the less critical yet nagging problems that affect everyday life (such as varicose veins, hemorrhoids or hay fever).

Orthomolecular doctors can be M.D.'s, D.O.'s, dentists or chiropractors. Orthomolecular doctors try to discover what is out of chemical balance in their patient's bodies and then try to fix it with nutrition. They recognize that nutritional healing may take longer and that sometimes traditional therapies such as drugs or surgery may be required.

"Most patients who come to an orthomolecular doctor have been the rounds with traditional medicine," says Richard P. Huemer, M.D., who is president of the Orthomolecular Medical Society, in Westlake Village, California. "Many have chronic degenerative diseases that have not yielded to conventional methods. But with proper nutrition and other natural methods, we usually achieve the desired results."

Naturopathic doctors are not M.D.'s or D.O.'s but receive an N.D. degree after completing a four-year program at a college of naturopathic medicine. "We're more into preventive medicine rather than crisis medicine," says Irvin H. Miller, N.D., president of the National Association of Naturopathic Physicians, in Tacoma, Washington, "and we believe in the healing power of nature. Our training teaches us to use nonpharmaceutical therapies such as spinal manipulation, acupuncture, homeopathic remedies, herbal treatments, hypnotherapy, biofeedback and massage. We're like family doctors of the old days.

"We use standard medical laboratory tests, too, but our margins for normal are much narrower. For example, most labs will use 50 to 120 as normal for a blood sugar," explains Dr. Miller. "But we use 85 to 100 as normal. We treat patients with chronic conditions such as arthritis, hypoglycemia, allergies, obesity, fatigue, poor digestion and much more. But we also recognize that there are certain conditions that we can't handle. We refer those patients to M.D.'s or D.O.'s."

Dentist, Endodontist, Orthodontist, Periodontist, Prosthodontist, Pedodontist and Oral Surgeon

Actually it is less complicated than you might think at first glance. That's because all of these specialists first had to become dentists, which means that all of them have earned a D.D.S. or D.M.D. degree. "Actually they are really the same thing," says James Berry of the American Dental Association. "It's just that some schools give the D.D.S. degree (doctor of dental surgery) while others give the D.M.D. degree (doctor of dental medicine). Either way, the student had to complete at least a four-year program of study at a dental college (most have a B.S. degree, too) before they could call themselves dentists. As for the specialties, each one involves five additional years of work to become certified—two years in the classroom and three years' experience in the field (except for oral surgery, which requires three of schooling and two in the field)."

So who do you go to for what? It's really easy. Ready? You'd take your kids to a *pedo*dontist. For braces you'd see an *ortho*dontist. Root-canal jobs are handled by an *endo*dontist. Gum problems are taken to a *perio*dontist. If it comes down to false teeth you'd go to a *prostho*dontist. And an oral surgeon takes care of anything requiring surgery—from impacted wisdom teeth to major reconstruction following an auto accident.

A regular dentist can do some of the basic work in all those areas too, but will refer you to a specialist if he feels he can't handle the problem.

Now does that clear up all your confusion? If not, don't be afraid to ask any health practitioner what his or her qualifications and experience are. You have a right to know. After all, it's your health and money.

CHAPTER 9

A Fresh Look at Chiropractic Care

It's not been easy for backache sufferers to decide which camp to try for relief: M.D. or D.C. (doctor of chiropractic). Chiropractors of yore were often placed in the same class as snake-oil salesmen, who stooped to any tactic to make a buck.

Chiropractors today are still somewhat painted by the same brush. M.D.'s claim there's no scientific evidence to support the chiropractors' claims of success, and that patients are at risk. D.C.'s maintain that chiropractic—a drugless, nonsurgical method of healing based on the premise that misaligned vertebrae, or subluxations, in the spine put pressure on spinal nerves and contribute to a variety of disorders—safely relieves pain. They say that their manual "adjustments" put things back in line and cause less harm than do the practices and pills used by M.D.'s.

Because of their sheer numbers and the prestige of the American Medical Association (AMA), the physicians' message usually overshadowed all else, and the chiropractors were left with the words "quack," "charlatan" and "cultist" ringing in their ears. They held on, though, and their patient rosters grew.

Several factors helped chiropractors gradually become entrenched in the medical field. One is the antitrust suit that several chiropractors filed against the AMA in 1976, charging the physicians' group with trying to prohibit free trade. The case is still tied up in court, but the

AMA has since stopped lumping chiropractors into the group's "unscientific cult" category.

Still another reason may be the rising number of backaches and the need for relief. It's estimated that seven million Americans are being treated for back pain, and new cases are being added at a rate of almost two million a year. Back pain is considered the most prevalent single medical ailment in the United States, with about $5 billion spent annually on diagnosis and treatment, not including compensation payments.

A Nation of Backaches

More than 20 million back operations are performed each year. But even some M.D.'s question the need for so much surgery, and the controversy over using the scalpel to heal backs has long been hotly debated within the AMA. Chiropractors point out that many patients adopt a what-have-I-got-to-lose attitude and give spinal manipulation a try before consenting to major surgery.

"Most of the people who come into my office have been to an M.D. first, and some are disillusioned or disappointed with the M.D.," says Milton Fried of Atlanta, who likens himself to a man without a country since he is both a licensed chiropractor and an M.D. "Patients aren't stupid. If they aren't getting relief from their pain, then they'll go somewhere else, and the success of chiropractic can be seen in the increasing number of patients."

At the turn of the decade, there were about nine million people seeing chiropractors, or roughly 4 percent of the U.S. population. A 1984 survey by the American Chiropractic Association (ACA) found that figure had risen to 10.7 million patients. More than 85 percent of the office visits were for neuromuscular problems, of which back and neck pain was the major symptom.

"The sophisticated consumer realizes there's a viable alternative to the traditional cure-the-disease approach to medicine that M.D.'s have been espousing and treating with drugs for years," says Louis Sportelli, D.C., and ACA board member and director of public affairs. "Chiropractic has been talking about the holistic, self-help aspects of health for years, things that people are just now starting to adopt. It's in vogue, and chiropractic's time is here."

Since the practice of adjusting spines first gained steam in 1895 when founding father D. D. Palmer opened the original school of chiropractic in Davenport, Iowa, there have been plenty of studies conducted by D.C.'s attesting to their success, which, of course, M.D.'s refused to consider credible.

Gaining Ground

Now, chiropractors point to the increasing number of reports that during the past decade have turned up on the pages of journals that physicians respect. Researchers from the University of Utah College of Medicine, for instance, reported that patients got as much satisfaction from chiropractors' treatment as they did from M.D.'s treatment. They contacted 232 persons who had been treated for back and spinal problems. Of these, 122 had been to D.C.'s and 110 had gone to M.D.'s. The scientists also tried to design the project to ensure that none of the participants held any prior animosity toward either type of practitioner.

While stressing the difficulty in comparing treatments, the authors did conclude that "chiropractors made patients feel better." ". . . the intervention of a chiropractor in problems (related to) neck and spine injuries was at least as effective as that of a physician, in terms of restoring the patient's function and satisfying the patient. . . ." (*Lancet,* June 29, 1974).

Canadian researchers report that while they can't conclude manipulation cures the cause of back pain in all cases, it definitely relieves suffering in the short term. Scientists at the University of Saskatchewan examined 283 people who were totally disabled by back pain. They were given a two- or three-week regimen of daily spinal manipulations by an experienced chiropractor and examined one month later and every three months thereafter.

"No patients were made worse by manipulation," they report, adding, "Most doctors, whether family physicians or surgeons, will wish to refer their patients to a practitioner of manipulative therapy. . . . The physician who makes use of this resource will provide relief for many back patients" (*Canadian Family Physician,* March, 1985).

A column in the March 20, 1980 edition of the *New England Journal of Medicine* dared suggest that physicians accept chiropractors as "limited medical practitioners," similar to optometrists, podiatrists

---

Chiropractors and X-Rays

You may not know exactly what to expect when first visiting a chiropractor, but one thing is usually certain: You'll have an x-ray.

Because chiropractic involves adjusting bones, no D.C. wants to put his hands on a patient until he knows the condition of that person's skeletal system. "It's a risk/benefit situation," says Louis Sportelli, D.C., an American Chiropractic Association spokesman. "The doctor and the patient take a big risk if the chiropractor makes any adjustments without knowing if there are any internal complications. If the patient is concerned about the exposure to radiation, he has to weigh the risks against the benefits and make a decision."

While some chiropractic opponents say D.C.'s take too many x-rays, Dr. Sportelli says his colleagues are aware of the hazards. "After the initial x-ray, it's usually a year before another is necessary because of the slow nature of structural changes. But if a patient comes in with a severe muscle spasm and is contorted, it may be necessary to do another in six to eight weeks, after he's straightened up and not in an odd position."

If you've recently seen other specialists who performed x-rays, ask for copies for the chiropractor. Also tell the D.C. if you are pregnant or if you've had any x-ray of any kind recently. You should also ask for a shield to protect reproductive organs.

---

or psychologists. Noting that "chiropractors appear to be winning their struggle to survive," the author also observes that "awareness of this fact is finally appearing in medical circles."

A research paper published in the *American Journal of Public Health* in July, 1982 stated that chiropractic is "the most popular form of nonmedical healing . . ." and "is an important source of care for many people." The author sidestepped the pros and cons of the debate, and avoided even giving a hint of a suggestion that M.D.'s make referrals to chiropractors, yet the conclusion is left to interpretation: "If it is felt that the use of medical facilities for some problems is inappropriate, then it may be in the physicians' and patients' best interest to promote a prescribed role for providers of alternative forms of health care."

Federal Findings

The federal government stepped into the fracas when a Congressional subcommittee asked the National Institutes of Health for "an independent, unbiased study" of chiropractic. A series of sessions were convened during the mid- to late-1970's at Michigan State University. The participants—Ph.D.'s, M.D.'s and D.O.'s—noted that most of the antichiropractor comments come from "those not trained in manipulative techniques," adding that data available at that time didn't clarify either position. "However, most participants . . . felt that manipulative therapy was of clinical value in the treatment of back pain."

The study that chiropractors found most satisfying emerged from New Zealand in 1979. A government-authorized commission of inquiry flatly stated that D.C.'s are experts in problems of the spine and M.D.'s are not, therefore "the medical practitioner, however skilled he may be in his particular field, is likely to miss what to a chiropractor would be obvious." The commission further reported that patients in the hands of registered chiropractors are safe, and that while chiropractors can't cure all ills, they are qualified to know when to refer cases to other specialists. "There is the clearest possible need for a closer degree of cooperation between doctors and chiropractors. . . . And now it has become plain that much medical criticism of chiropractors is based on simple ignorance of what they do. . . ."

There's also an increasing body of empirical evidence, such as the fact that more insurance organizations are covering chiropractic care costs. Medicare, which wouldn't touch chiropractic bills until 1972, now covers a very limited portion, while a number of states allow payments through Medicaid. Payments are also made through worker's compensation. Blue Cross and Blue Shield, one of the nation's largest insurers, now provides coverage in 26 states, with action pending elsewhere, according to a spokesperson. The organization has no national policy regarding coverage, with decisions based on the situation or laws in each state.

Wading into the Mainstream

There are other signs that chiropractors are getting into mainstream medicine. About half a dozen hospitals now have D.C.'s on staff. More chiropractors and M.D.'s are cutting deals for partnerships in private practice, which, according to Dr. Fried, is common in larger cities. Of the 18 chiropractic colleges, 16 have met federal accreditation standards.

To chiropractors, one of the most telling signs of the times came when the AMA in 1979 rescinded its canon that forbade members from referring patients to D.C.'s The AMA offers no reason for its action, although chiropractors believe the antitrust suit had a lot to do with it. The AMA official stance can be found in its code of ethics, which states that there is no scientific evidence that spinal manipulation can help ailments such as hypertension and heart disease. But it doesn't rule out the possibility that chiropractic may offer some therapeutic value, "nor does it mean that all chiropractors should be equated with cultists." An M.D. may refer a patient to any licensed practitioner whenever "this will benefit the patient."

Even with the subtle signs that the haze of confusion may be clearing somewhat, it still could be perplexing for some people to decide whether they should take their aches to a chiropractor. Those who do opt in favor of a D.C. will soon realize that the selection process is just as difficult as it is for choosing an M.D. Until you've been treated a few times, it's hard to tell whether you made the right choice.

You can tell something about a D.C.'s philosophy and treatment by his affiliation with one of the three national chiropractic organizations:

• The American Chiropractic Association (ACA), the largest with more than 17,000 members, generally consists of the liberal practitioners who use manipulation plus other techniques that may include massage, vitamin therapy, special diets, exercise, ultrasound, vibrators, colonic irrigation or even acupuncture.

• The Internal Chiropractors Association (ICA) represents about 8,000 of the more conservative ("straight") practitioners who may at times offer nutrition and exercise advice, but whose primary focus is adjusting the spine, says executive director Bruce Nordstrom, D.C.

• The Federation of Straight Chiropractors is the smallest group, claiming a few thousand "superstraight" members and strongly holding to the belief that D.C.'s should be adjusters of the spine only. Says board chairman Joseph Donofrio, D.C., "Our members are competent chiropractors who aren't therapists, they only adjust spines." Two colleges educate D.C.'s who adhere to this belief, and the Federation supports the SCASA (Straight Chiropractic Academic Standards Association), whose accreditation standards differ from the ACA and ICA educational criteria.

A Weighty Decision

When considering whether to go to one of the three types of D.C.'s or even an M.D., base the decision on personal need and belief, says Dr. Fried, who's been on both sides of the fence. "It depends on how that person feels about his health. If you have no problem with taking drugs for almost every illness or condition, go to a physician. If you want an alternative, try a chiropractor. The patient needs to be aware of what each has to offer, and then make a decision. Neither knows it all, and if one claims he does, the patient should get up and leave immediately. For the best all-around health care, a person might consider going to both."

Dr. Donofrio warns that "anyone who says they can cure cancer or heart disease or similar problems, they are the real quacks. They are trouble for patients and are the ones who have helped give chiropractors a negative image." (So far 40 states have provisions to revoke the licenses of unethical chiropractors, with actions pending in several other states.)

All three spokesmen for the D.C. organizations agree that patients should be wary of a chiropractor who flatly refuses to consider referring a problem to an M.D. "And vice versa," says Dr. Sportelli. "Medical doctors should be willing to put ego aside and refer a patient for the sake of the patient's health."

The easiest way to tell whether the time has come to switch healers is to pose to yourself a simple question: Does it still hurt? "No one's going to continue suffering for long just because a doctor tells them that it will be all right someday. It may often take a little while to start feeling better because neither an M.D. nor chiropractor can cure everything overnight, but patients won't wait forever. They'll go where they can get relief," says Dr. Fried.

It's Multiple Choice for Backache Sufferers

The choice for a back-pain victim is not merely between an M.D.'s "drugs and surgery" and a chiropractor's manipulation. Many medical physicians, even orthopedic surgeons, prescribe therapeutic exercise and physical therapy to prevent the need for surgery. Back-pain clinics, which may be staffed by M.D.'s, therapists, nurses and health educators, typically offer a variety of approaches. One recent study of back pain gave especially high grades to a little known branch of medicine known as physiatry (fizz-EYE-a-tree), whose practitioners are M.D.'s with advanced training in physical medicine. And many osteopathic physicians, though licensed to prescribe drugs or perform surgery, may use manipulation as a first resort, though their technique is not the same as a chiropractor's.

Chiropractic is therefore one alternative among many.

CHAPTER 10

Medical Jargon: Can *You* Decipher It?

Ever wonder why doctors say clavicle instead of collarbone, and diaphoresis instead of sweat? Or why they sometimes throw around words like idiopathic, antipyretic or contraindicated? When you walk out of your doctor's office can you honestly say you understood everything he told you? If you don't, you're not alone. Call it medicalese, medibabble or medispeak, it still comes out the same—confusing.

According to two language specialists, jargon has proved convenient to politicians, bureaucrats, lawyers, educators, physicians and others because it conceals fuzzy thinking while projecting an illusion of wisdom. "Mysterious-sounding words are often so intimidating they ward off any challenges from listeners," says Lois DeBakey, Ph.D., and Selma DeBakey, professors of scientific communication at Baylor College of Medicine, in Houston.

Doctors who use unnecessary jargon (which the professors call "medicant") "rely on the uncritical acceptance of their words by their audiences." Let's face it, "few people are courageous or secure enough to ask a doctor to translate ominous scientific terms into plain English," say the DeBakeys. Yet incomprehensive language ill-serves the user. It "drives a wedge between the medical community and the rest of the public; it creates an image of aloofness, impersonality, smugness and indifference"—traits the DeBakeys think most doctors don't have. More important, they add, "it perverts the purpose of language—communication—by creating confusion, ambiguity, misinterpretation, inadvertent humor or sheer tedium. If patients misunderstand the physician's explanation, they may become tense, apprehensive or depressed; if they misinterpret instructions, they will be unable to cooperate effectively in their treatment."

You can avoid those problems by becoming fluent in medicalese yourself. It's not as difficult as you might imagine, and learning some of the jargon just may give you the confidence you need to speak up to your doctor. Begin by taking this medical quiz, selecting the word or phrase that best describes each term. You may find out that you already know more doctor-talk than you thought.

1. ADIPOSE
   a. fatty
   b. additional x-rays
   c. totaling the bill
   answer: a. You may hear this word used more often in the phrase "adipose tissue." It refers to the layer of connective tissue beneath the skin that contains many fat cells. The more overweight you are, the more adipose tissue you have.

2. AMBULATORY
   a. transported by ambulance
   b. able to walk
   c. unable to walk
   answer: b. In spite of the way this word sounds, being ambulatory is actually good.

3. ANALGESIC
   a. painkiller
   b. rectal medicine
   c. antibiotic
   answer: a. When your doctor says to take a mild analgesic he means aspirin or perhaps acetaminophen (a nonaspirin pain reliever). Actually the word breaks down into *an,* meaning "no," and *algesis,* which means "pain."

4. ANTIPYRETIC
   a. bleeding gums

b. antacid

c. fever reducer

answer: c. When you break this word down you get *anti,* meaning "against," and *pyr,* meaning "fire." Aspirin or acetaminophen are the most commonly used antipyretics.

5. ATROPHY

a. prize for best patient

b. weight loss

c. shrinkage (of muscle or other tissue)

answer: c. This wasting away of tissue usually occurs with a lack of use. You may have noticed muscular atrophy if you've ever had a cast on an arm or leg for several months. That's because those muscles were totally immobilized during that time. Of course this type of atrophy is temporary and the muscles regain their original strength.

Unfortunately, atrophy can also be a symptom of more serious disorders.

6. BENIGN

a. noncancerous

b. fast-growing

c. cancerous

answer: a. If you hear the doctor say benign, heave a sigh of relief. This is good news. On the other hand, malignant means cancerous. For some reason, patients confuse these words and assign the scary meaning to benign.

7. CONGENITAL

a. friendly disposition

b. a disorder of the genitals

c. condition present at birth

answer: c. A congenital disorder means that you didn't contract it from a germ—like a cold. This is something that developed before you were even born, such as a congenital heart defect.

8. CONTRAINDICATED

a. recommended

b. to be avoided

c. makes no difference

answer: b. If your doctor says that estrogen replacement therapy is contraindicated for someone with a family history of cancer, he means don't take it.

9. DERMATITIS
   a. tight skin
   b. inflammation of the skin
   c. numbness of the skin
   answer: b. Remember this hint. Whenever a word ends in *itis,* it means "inflammation." In the case of dermatitis, that's actually a catchall phrase for any skin irritation in which there is redness, itching and rash.

10. EDEMA
   a. swelling
   b. pertaining to an enema
   c. bruising
   answer: a. This is a condition in which the tissues contain an excessive amount of fluid. It's common to see edema in the ankles and feet of women in the later stages of pregnancy, for example. But it could also signal a problem in kidney function.

11. ETIOLOGY
   a. the study of eating
   b. the study of nutrition
   c. pertaining to the causes of disease
   answer: c. You may see this word written more often than spoken, but either way it's simply a sophisticated way of discussing the cause of an illness.

12. FEBRILE
   a. high in fiber
   b. feverish
   c. weak
   answer: b. If your doctor says you are in a febrile state, he means that you also have the symptoms that accompany a rise in temperature: headache, pains, loss of appetite and a general, all-over discomfort.

13. HEMATOMA
   a. bruise

b. broken toe

c. iron deficiency

answer: a. Here's a fancy way to say you've got a black-and-blue mark. And most of the time it's as innocuous as that. But depending on where the hematoma is, it could mean big trouble. Ben Casey (the former TV neurosurgeon) often had patients with subdural hematomas. That's a bruise in the brain as a result of a blow to the head. More likely, your hematomas are due to bumping into furniture.

14. HEMORRHAGE

    a. bleeding

    b. pertaining to hemorrhoids

    c. old blood

    answer: a. You may think that a hemorrhage always refers to an enormous flow of blood ("he suffered a massive hemorrhage") but in fact even minor bleeding can be called a hemorrhage.

15. IDIOPATHIC

    a. of lower intelligence

    b. not able to walk a straight line

    c. of unknown cause

    answer: c. Any time a doctor uses this word to preface the name of a disease, he is simply telling you that they don't know what causes it.

    Meanwhile, you're probably thinking the worst. Sometimes, doctors may use "essential" instead, as in "essential hypertension." But it means the same thing as idiopathic.

16. LESION

    a. any sore or wound

    b. a group of health practitioners

    c. relief from stress

    answer: a. Here's another catchall word that covers everything from skin sores associated with eczema to the lung damage in tuberculosis. Even ulcers, tumors and cataracts can be called lesions.

17. NEGATIVE TEST RESULT

    a. the patient has the disorder

    b. the patient doesn't have the disorder

    c. the patient died

answer: b. Here's a case where less is more, since negative test results indicate normal.

On the other hand, a positive test result could mean bad news. For example, if your blood sugar result is positive, it could mean diabetes.

18. PARENTERAL
    a. disease inherited from parents
    b. medicine given by parents
    c. medicine given by injection
    answer: c. This looks for sure like it has something to do with parents. But of course it doesn't. It just means not by mouth. So when a medicine is given parenterally, it means not in pill form but by injection.

19. PROGNOSIS
    a. disease of the nose
    b. a chronic condition
    c. expected outcome of a disease
    answer: c. This sounds just like any other disease ending in *osis,* such as cirrh*osis* or artheroscler*osis*. But it isn't. It literally means foreknowledge. So if your doctor says "the prognosis is good," he expects you to recover.

20. PRURITIS
    a. infection producing pus
    b. itching
    c. of highest purity
    answer: b. Why can't they just say itching if that's what they mean, especially since "pruritis" sounds similar to "purulent," a word that means "pus-forming"?

21. PSYCHOGENIC
    a. of unsound mind
    b. having an emotional origin
    c. having a genetic origin
    answer: b. Some headaches may be psychogenic disorders if they are caused by emotional upset or stress. Asthma and colitis can also fall into the psychogenic category. But not appendicitis or a toothache.

22. Q.I.D.
    a. take four times a day

b. take for four days

c. "quit if disagreeable"

answer: a. Now you know what those letters on your prescription mean. Actually they stand for the Latin "quater in die." If it says t.i.d. instead, then it means take three times a day ("ter in die"); b.i.d. ("bis in die") means twice a day.

23. SEPSIS

a. infection

b. cleanliness

c. waste removal

answer: a. This kind of infection refers to the presence in your system of bacteria or their poisons. If you eat contaminated foods, for example, the doctor may say you're having an attack of intestinal sepsis.

24. SEQUELA

a. aftereffect of a disease

b. quiet atmosphere

c. food poisoning

answer: a. Think of "sequel" and you've got the answer. In medicine, when a second disorder develops as a direct result of the first one, it's called a "sequela." For example, rheumatic fever is a sequela of a strep throat infection. And the deadly Reye's syndrome may be a sequela of a common viral infection.

25. SUBCLINICAL

a. the basement of the hospital

b. a poorly equipped hospital

c. having no visible symptoms

answer: c. Refers to the period before the appearance of typical symptoms of a disease. In other words, when you're only a little bit sick, the doctor may say you have a subclinical case of the disease.

26. SUBCUTANEOUS

a. not very pretty

b. beneath the skin

c. underfed

answer: b. You're most likely to hear this word when your doctor is ordering an injection of medicine. He means that the drug should be administered just below the skin.

27. SYNDROME
    a. infected sinusues
    b. a recurring infection
    c. a specific collection of symptoms
    answer: c. The grouping of symptoms always indicates a particular disease or abnormal condition and helps the doctor in the diagnosis. Some of the more common ones are alcohol withdrawal syndrome, Reye's syndrome, restless legs syndrome and sudden infant death syndrome, but there are many others.

28. SYSTEMIC
    a. affecting the whole body
    b. methodical
    c. cyst forming
    answer: a. If your doctor says he's giving you a systemic remedy, he means it's a drug that will work on the whole body.

29. TOPICAL
    a. overheated
    b. on the surface
    c. pertinent discussion
    answer: b. A medicine applied topically simply means that it is to be spread (as in an ointment) on a specific area of the skin surface and will affect only that area.

30. URTICARIA
    a. hives
    b. burping
    c. standing upright
    answer: a. Usually from an allergic reaction to foods, drugs, emotional stress or insect bites.

Scoring

Give yourself one point for each correct answer. If you scored:

24-30—You're already well versed in medispeak and because of that you rarely misunderstand your doctor's explanations or instructions.

12-23—You're on your way to fluency but you still need some assistance. That's why you often ask your doctor to explain the words you are unfamiliar with even though it sometimes makes you feel a little uncomfortable.

0-11—You need to invest in a medical dictionary for lay people—and use it. Only then will you be able to change your feelings of intimidation to those of self-confidence.

CHAPTER 11

Is the Price Right?

You come down with pneumonia, land in a hospital for a few days, then later get the bill in the mail: $6,230.

With that kind of money you could buy a new car or a month-long romp on the French Riviera. There must be some mistake.

No mistake. According to unpublished Medicare data, $6,230 is the average hospital charge for treatment of prolonged respiratory infections.

Despite all the headlines about stampeding health-care costs, the problem never seems completely real until it rampages through your own bank account. You read the medical bill and go into price-tag shock (PTS), a condition marked by bug eyes, a dropped jaw and the realization that everything from pacemakers to penicillin costs real dollars.

Having health insurance or Medicare can deter this realization for a while, but sooner or later the bad news sets in. Like when your medical coverage won't stretch far enough to blot out the bills—or as is often the case with Medicare—your coverage shrinks.

The cure for price-tag shock, of course, is price-tag awareness (PTA)—knowing more about the costs of getting well. Such knowledge allows you to be more selective about certain health-care services, encourages you to look for ways to cut costs and helps you guard against billing errors and overcharging.

To test your PTA—and to give prices of some medical treatments and tests—we offer this quiz. (Most of the prices shown are averages, and medical charges can vary with the doctor, hospital and area involved. And even though the figures are based on recent information, in some cases they may not be absolutely current. So some of the costs presented may actually be even higher.)

1. Your family practitioner charges you $50 for a complete history and physical exam. Is his fee in line with prevailing rates?

Yes: $50 is the median charge for family practitioners. The median for general practitioners is $44; for internists, $76.

2. Who charges more for first office visits, city or country doctors?

The median charge is consistently higher for city physicians, regardless of their type of practice. The median fee for urban family practitioners, for example, is $26. For their rural counterparts, $21.

3. You slip on the ice, fracture your hip and end up in the hospital. Your hospital bill matches the national average and is (a) under $2,000, (b) under $3,000 or (c) over $4,000.

Answer: (c). The average hospital stay for a fractured hip is 17 days at a cost of $4,144.

4. Your doctor prescribes the antibiotic amoxicillin for a respiratory infection you have. If you could buy the drug wholesale, a month's supply could cost as much as (a) $10, (b) $32 or (c) $47?

Answer: (b). The retail, or drugstore, price could be far higher.

5. The average cost of having a baby in a hospital delivery room is approximately (a) $1,200, (b) $1,800 or (c) $2,100?

Answer: (c). And this price doesn't include the anesthesiologist's fee, which averages $64. If the baby is delivered cesarean, the average cost goes up to $3,340.

6. In which city does it cost more to have a total hysterectomy, (a) Los Angeles, (b) Atlanta, (c) Chicago or (d) Dallas.

Answer: (a). The average surgical charges in L.A. is $1,634. In Atlanta it's $1,078; in Chicago, $1,324; in Dallas, $1,186. But the highest average charge for this procedure is found in New York City: $1,922. The national average is more like $1,141.

7. The artificial heart implanted in William J. Schroeder, the second human recipient of such a device, cost (a) $55,000, (b) $500,000 or (c) $45,000?

Answer: (a). The implanted unit cost $15,000, and its drive system cost $40,000.

8. Which costs more, a vasectomy or a tubal sterilization?

Tubal sterilizations cost nearly five times more than vasectomies, the former averaging $1,180 and the latter averaging $241. The cost difference is due in part to the hospital charges involved in most tubal procedures.

9. Which surgical procedure costs the most, (a) appendectomy, (b) hemorrhoidectomy, (c) gallbladder removal or (d) tonsillectomy?

Answer: (c). The average surgeon's fees are $637 for appendectomy; $405, hemorrhoidectomy; $936, gallbladder removal; and $370, tonsillectomy.

10. Which dental fee is way above the national average, (a) porcelain crown with gold, $304, (b) initial oral exam, $24, (c) permanent amalgam filling, $31 or (d) complete lower dentures, $340?

Answer: (b). The average charges for an initial oral exam is only $12.

11. Which contraceptive method costs the least, (a) the Pill, (b) IUD, (c) condom, (d) foam or (e) diaphragm?

Answer: (c). The average first-year cost for the condom method is $30. The most expensive form of contraception is the Pill, with a first-year cost of $172.

12. Which state has the highest average charge for a one-day stay in a semiprivate hospital room, (a) Pennsylvania, (b) South Carolina, (c) California or (d) Oregon?

Answer: (c). California's rate is $276 per day, but the highest in the nation is Washington D.C.'s, with $285. The lowest is found in South Carolina, with $136. The national average is $203.

13. You have your first heart attack. If your hospital bill is average, will it be about (a) $2,100, (b) $3,500 or (c) $5,300?

Answer: (c). The charge is for an average stay of ten days.

14. You're having fainting spells, and no one knows why. How much will it cost you to get a definitive diagnosis of your condition?

Far more than you think. A recent study of people who fainted for unknown reasons revealed that the average cost for their evaluation and hospitalization was $2,463. Yet in only 11 percent of the cases could doctors find a cause for the fainting.

15. Who has the highest median charge for office visits (other than the first one), (a) family practitioners, (b) plastic surgeons, (c) obstetrician-gynecologists or (d) pediatricians?

Answer: (c). The median fee among Ob-Gyns is $25.

16. The average surgical fee for a radical mastectomy is (a) $1,147, (b) $3,215 or (c) $4,405?

Answer: (a). The average charge is higher in major cities than in nonmetropolitan areas. Fees average $1,423 in Dallas, for example, but $856 in southern Indiana.

17. Iatrogenic diseases are those conditions *caused by* medical treatment, and apparently they are more prevalent than most people believe. What's the average hospital bill for treating iatrogenic problems, (a) $32, (b) $113, (c) $3,517 or (d) $4,208?

Answer: (c).

18. The average hospital bill for dilatation and curettage (D & C) is (a) $755, (b) $1,378 or (c) $1,632?

Answer: (b). The procedure involves an average hospital stay of 3.6 days.

19. Your ophthalmologist gives you a comprehensive eye exam and charges you $65. Is his fee out of line with prevailing rates?

The charge is well within bounds. The national average cost for a one-hour ophthalmological exam is $70 to $85.

20. You enter the hospital to have plastic surgery done on your nose. Your total bill (including surgeon's fee and room and board) is average. Is it (a) $714, (b) $910, (c) $1,276 or (d) $1,399?

Answer: d. The procedure involves an average hospital stay of 3.4 days.

21. You fracture your thighbone in a skiing accident, and you have to spend time in the hospital. Your treatment and length of stay are typical. The bill comes to (a) $640, (b) $1,450, (c) $5,300 or (d) $10,250?

Answer: (c). The average stay is 22.7 days.

22. Two simple test for urinary tract infections, the nitrite test and the leukocyte test, are available in many drugstores for $1 or less. A laboratory urinalysis may cost as much as (a) $5, (b) $10, (c) $20 or (d) $25?

Answer: (d).

23. Which carries the highest price tag, (a) heart transplant, (b) treatment of extensive burns or (c) coronary bypass?

Answer: (b). The total average hospital bill for major burn treatment is $26,180; for heart transplant, $19,118; and for bypass, $15,676.

CHAPTER 12

Walk-In Doctoring: The New Health-Care Option

It's Sunday evening and that respiratory infection you've been battling all week has just called up reinforcements. It's germ warfare, and your body's losing.

Think fast: Should you call your doctor? You can't. His hours are 9 to 5, weekdays only. Should you drive to the hospital emergency room? Wrong. It's 20 miles away and three times as expensive as your family physician. Besides, the last time you were there you had to wait four hours while the medical team sewed up crash victims and screened drug addicts.

You've got it: You'll zip down to the shopping mall and pop into the walk-in medical center. You'll be diagnosed, treated and back home in 30 minutes flat.

Walk-in medical center? It sounds like something that's been around ever since physicians stopped making house calls, but walk-in centers offering all-around doctoring are about as newfangled as you can get in American health care.

To the dismay of many private practitioners and the delight of thousands of patients, walk-in medical centers (often called freestanding emergency centers) have evolved into a whole new breed of medical practice—a cross between the family physician and the hospital emergency room. Like your local M.D., the centers treat pains, fevers, cuts and breaks (everything but life-threatening emergencies). And like an emergency room, they have extended hours (most are open 12 to 14 hours per day) and no appointments.

And don't look now, but such a novelty may have just cropped up in your neighborhood. There are over 1,100 of them coast to coast, and they're opening up at the rate of at least one a day. This year probably as many as 25 million people will bypass family doctors and hospital emergency rooms to get medical help in these centers, and next year the numbers are likely to be larger.

The force behind the trend is easy enough to identify, say the advocates of walk-in medicine: The centers exist because people need and want them.

"People don't use health care the way they used to," says James R. Roberts, executive director of the National Association of Freestanding Emergency Centers. "The consumer now demands medical treatment that's more accessible and more affordable, and these centers help meet those requirements."

"There' a clear need for convenient, consumer-oriented quality care," says Joseph G. Maloney, M.D., vice-president of a chain of walk-in centers in the Boston area. "In no other industry is the relationship between the consumer and the provider as unbalanced as in health care. You wait for a week for an appointment, and then the average waiting time in a doctor's office is one hour. If the doctor's office is closed, you go to the emergency room and wait until the life-and-death emergency cases are taken care of. Any dry cleaner that operated this way would be put out of business."

Freestanding Care in Boston

Critics of the centers, on the other hand, see them as an awkward step in precisely the wrong direction. They believe that walk-in clinics probably provide questionable health care ("Docs-in-a-Box" and "7-Eleven Medicine" are favorite epithets), and that they break up the "continuity of care" offered by family doctors.

True or false? It may be too early to tell. But we think we uncovered some clues when we took a firsthand look at Dr. Maloney's half dozen walk-ins that dot the Boston suburbs.

Called Health Stop, they have all the consumer conveniences that their slick moniker implies. Scrubbed and spacious facilities (with examination rooms, waiting areas, conference rooms, x-ray rooms, even children's play areas) announce themselves where the people are—suburban thoroughfares and shopping centers. At each clinic, two full-time doctors and about ten full- or part-time nurses and medical assistants treat patients without appointments seven days a week, 8 A.M. to 9 P.M. And they do so with impressive efficiency: Patients are greeted within 30 seconds after they walk through the door and are seen by a doctor within 15 minutes.

"Patients seem to like what we're doing here," says C. Matthew Masserman, M.D., medical director at one of the centers. "So far, feedback from patients has been almost all positive."

Other Health Stop physicians report much the same. And considering the wide spectrum of care the doctors offer, such blessings from their patients may be some kind of record.

"We're a doctor's office with extended capabilities," says Dr. Maloney. "People can come to us because they have a sore throat or fracture or want a physical exam, and we can diagnose swiftly because we have laboratory and x-ray equipment on the premises. We practice general medicine with a consumerist twist."

What they don't do, however, is pretend to be an emergency room capable of handling crises that threaten life and limb. And neither do most other walk-in medical centers. Like other walk-ins, Health Stop clinics don't accept ambulances. And the word "emergency" (used warily in half the other 1,100 walk-ins) has become a no-no among Health Stop's marketing and medical personnel.

It's just as well. The word, and the idea it conveys, has been the focus of criticism of walk-in centers everywhere. Some physicians charge that, whether or not "emergency" is on a walk-in's shingle, it's too easy for a critically ill patient to run to a walk-in medical center when he should be hurrying to a hospital emergency room. The detour, they say, could be fatal.

Doctors at walk-ins counter that they go out of their way to help people make the distinction between the two kinds of care. Besides, they say, if somebody with a life-threatening medical emergency does show up at the door, they're trained and equipped to stabilize him and transport him to the hospital.

"Like most other walk-in centers," says Dr. Maloney, "each Health Stop is equipped with oxygen gear, defibrillator, crash cart [mobile emergency medicine chest], monitors and more. We're ready for serious medical problems should they arise. And once in a while they do arise, just as they do in a doctor's office. The difference is we're ready, and some doctors' offices aren't."

More Than Meets the Eye

How walk-in medical centers handle more routine health problems, though, may be a better test of the quality of their care. At Health Stop, at least, there are signs that the analogies to fast-food stores are wide of the mark.

"We've taken steps to ensure that the consumer gets his money's worth," Dr. Maloney says. "We've staffed the centers with the most qualified physicians we could find. We make sure that all x-rays and cardiograms are double-checked by radiologists and cardiologists. Four of our centers are affiliated with hospitals to augment our medical services. And every month we submit staff doctors to a rigorous review by a committee of their peers. The committee ensures that doctors aren't overtesting or overmedicating, that they're treating patients correctly and consistently."

Critics of convenience-store medicine might find a peculiar irony here. Health Stop's emphasis on efficiency and consumerism (strange notions to a lot of traditional doctors) is the very thing that seems to propel the staff doctors toward a more human approach to patients.

"I think we're more likely to view patients from a holistic perspective," says Dr. Maloney. "We advise them on preventive health measures, on lifestyle changes that can have a positive effect on their health. It's because we want patients to come back again. If all we did was bandage people up without taking an interest in their attitudes and habits, we would soon lose those patients. They could go elsewhere for bandaging, but there are few places where they could get this extra dimension to treatment."

"There's time to practice preventive medicine here," says Dr. Masserman. "An efficient management firm takes care of Health Stop's business and financial chores, so staff physicians can devote 100 percent of their time to treating and advising patients. We're even showing our nurses how to teach people about specific diets, high blood pressure, medication and other things they should know about."

Despite such amenities, are the centers fragmenting the traditional relationship between patient and family practitioner? And are patients getting lost in the centers' well-greased mechanisms of health care?

Conventional practitioners have always maintained that people get the best health care from family doctors who know them well and see them year after year. And few health-care experts would disagree. This ideal arrangement, however, may not entirely match up with reality. Up to 35 percent of adults, for example, don't have a family physician.

"Despite the present surplus of doctors," says Dr. Maloney, "many people refuse to interact with the traditional medical system. So health care is already fragmented in this country. What we're doing is providing a reasonable alternative for people who aren't interested in the old system."

And judging from reports of both patients and staff, no one has yet been misplaced in the Health Stop shuffle. "We follow up on all patients 24 hours after we see them," says an emergency-medicine specialist at one of the centers. "We call them to tell them laboratory results, to see how they're feeling. And when we refer them to a specialist, we make the appointment for them and follow up later."

When 40-year-old Patricia Storella got something in her left eye, she thought the pain and redness would go away in a couple of hours. When it didn't, she walked down to the Health Stop center in Medford, and the doctor on duty saw her in less than 10 minutes. And in another 20 minutes he had examined her eye, flushed out the foreign matter and sent her on her way. "The amazing thing was," she says, "they not only took care of the problem right away, they called me back the next day to check on me. Their follow-up is impressive."

The cost of all the TLC may eventually become Health Stop's biggest selling point. Like most walk-in medical centers, Health Stop's fees are comparable to those of family physicians and dramatically lower than emergency-room charges. (The average bill at a walk-in is $48 to $50.) At Health Stop clinics, fees are 30 to 40 percent of the average fee in emergency rooms.

And it stands to reason. Emergency rooms by design are facilities with high overhead. They're open around the clock, they're sometimes overstaffed, they have to buy and use a lot of expensive lifesaving equipment. It's therefore fairly easy to walk into one with a sore throat and leave with a bill for $100.

"Walk-in medical centers are a welcome reversal of the trend toward high-priced health care," says Dr. Maloney. "In most areas of technology, products and services start out relatively expensive (like transistor radios and video equipment) and gradually get more economical as development proceeds. But the exact opposite happens in medical care. We think people will be encouraged to come to our centers because we're not part of this upward spiral."

It will be the consumer who passes down the final verdict on walk-in care. And judging from consumer reaction thus far, centers like Health Stop have nothing to worry about.

CHAPTER 13

Medical Tests: Don't Bet Your Life on Them

The last time you went to the doctor's, more than likely he took your blood pressure. With a hand-held rubber bulb, he inflated a cuff wrapped around your bicep, placed a stethoscope over the artery near your elbow, and then listened as he slowly release the air pressure. The moment he began to hear a tapping sound (your pulse), he noted the height of a column of mercury in a tall glass tube connected to the cuff. That was your systolic pressure (at your heart's contracting phase). As the cuff deflated still further, the tapping sound grew louder, then changed suddenly to very soft, then completely disappeared. At the moment the sound vanished, he noted the mercury's height a second time. That was your diastolic (relaxing phase) pressure.

And there you have it: one of the simplest, most common tests in medicine. Yet, for various reasons, the results of this test may have fallen outside an acceptable margin of error—or even been grossly inaccurate. For one thing, just being there in the doctor's office getting tested is enough to falsely elevate most people's blood pressure. For another, unless the equipment your doctor was using had been regularly serviced, the readings it gave him may well have been unreliable.

In an effort to test the accuracy and working condition of these devices (called sphygmomanometers) in actual practice, a scientific team examined 310 of them being used in seven Michigan hospitals. They found that almost a third of them deviated from normal by a significant margin; nearly 19 percent of these were seriously in error. "Significant errors in blood-pressure classification, risk appraisal and clinical management could be made from these spurious [incorrect] values," the scientists noted (*Archives of Internal Medicine,* June, 1970).

In another survey, 210 sphygmomanometers in hospitals and doctors' offices in Ireland were examined. Faults in the inflation/deflation system, caused mainly by dirt and wear, were found to be common; leakage was found in 48 percent of the hospital machines and 33 percent of those in private practices. Thirty percent of one model gave seriously misleading readings. And 94 percent of all the machines had cuff widths shorter than the length recommended for normal use on adults (*British Medical Journal,* August 14, 1982).

A false reading on a blood pressure test may not strike you as a major tragedy (though it *can* have a significant effect on later treatment). But what about a test that fails to catch a cancerous tumor in your lung at a stage when it's still operable, or tells you that you've got diabetes, hypoglycemia or dangerously elevated serum cholesterol . . . when you don't? Very few medical tests are infallible, and for some, the known margin of error is astonishingly wide.

The sheer number of medical tests performed each year in the United States is staggering: In 1981, according to government reports, 10 *billion* tests were done. That's roughly 40 tests per person. The total bill for all this testing, from x-rays and stress tests to analyses of urine and blood (there are 850 different tests on blood alone), came to about $140 billion dollars, or nearly the total tab for health care.

Yet a number of scientists estimate that as many as 15 percent of the most common lab tests are either slightly or seriously in error. Though this estimate has been hotly disputed by pathologists, things are better than they used to be: In 1964, Centers for Disease Control (CDC) director David Spencer, M.D., estimated that up to 25 percent of all laboratory test results were unreliable.

Even so, if a 15 percent estimate is right, that means something like one out of every seven tests comes back from the lab bearing data that is misleading or simply wrong. That's four million erroneous test results *each day.*

Errors can creep into the testing procedure in a variety of ways. The equipment used to perform the test may be poorly maintained, as in the case of sphygmomanometers. Lab technicians may be careless or lack proper training. Or the test itself, even if poorly administered, may leave a great deal to be desired.

"Most old, outmoded tests do not die; they rarely—regardless of their costs or value—even fade away," write Cathey Pinckney and Edward R. Pinckney, M.D., in their book, *The Encyclopedia of Medical Tests* (Facts on File). A good example is the stress electrocardiogram, says Dr. Pinckney. It's administered while the patient runs or walks on a treadmill, climbs steps or performs other vigorous exercise; it's meant to show potential heart damage as well as previously undetected minimal heart damage.

Yet, more than 50 percent of the time, the test fails to show these abnormalities in patients who have them, Dr. Pinckney says. (That's a failure of the test's *sensitivity,* or ability to detect disease states when they're actually present.) What's more, when the stress test is given to those with no heart disease at all, more than half get false positive results, indicating they *do* have some pathology. (That's a failure of the test's *specificity,* or the degree to which it falsely indicates the presence of disease where none exists.) A test's sensitivity and specificity, taken together, make up its *predictive value,* or relative accuracy. In the case of the stress electrocardiogram, its relative accuracy is dismally low.

Testing for cholesterol levels in the blood is another procedure with a very low level of accuracy. "It's probably one of the most inaccurate individual tests we have to do," Dr. Pinckney told us. "If I said, 'tsk, tsk,' while taking a sample of blood for cholesterol analysis, I could raise your cholesterol 20 points."

X-Rays for Cancer: 30 Percent Error Rate

By their very nature, some tests are just not very precise; they force physicians to peer "through a glass, darkly." X-ray screening for lung cancer is another good example. Over the years, studies have repeatedly shown that 20 to 50 percent of detectable malignant tumors are completely missed, detected but not reported, or reported but misinterpreted when they first appear on x-rays. These are serious errors, because they delay diagnosis and treatment and therefore reduce the patient's chances of survival.

One study examined the decisions that led to such errors in 27 cases of lung cancer. In 22 cases, the tumor's ominous shadow was simply missed on the x-rays. In four cases, they were noticed but misinterpreted. And in one case, there were errors in both detection and interpretation of the x-ray results. Though the one proven method of reducing the error rate in lung-cancer diagnosis is having a second specialist examine the x-rays, "over 90 percent of our errors involved cases in which roentgenograms [x-rays] were reviewed by more than one radiologist.

"An error rate of about 30 percent appears to be an unavoidable aspect of chest radiology as it is currently practiced," the researchers conclude (*Western Journal of Medicine,* June, 1981). Because of the known limits of accuracy in x-ray screening, they add, radiologists should not be held legally responsible for missing or misinterpreting an x-ray shadow caused by lung cancer.

Glucose-Tolerance Test: Questionable Results

The glucose-tolerance test, which for years has been considered the best means of diagnosing diabetes, is another test of doubtful accuracy. In fact, most Americans diagnosed as diabetic don't have diabetes and never will, says Marvin D. Siperstein, M.D., professor of medicine at the University of California, San Francisco, School of Medicine.

"This is probably the grossest example of overdiagnosis in medicine," Dr. Siperstein told a nutrition seminar. "And wait until the lawyers get hold of the fact that over one half of people treated with oral agents in this country aren't diabetic" (*Internal Medicine News,* September 1, 1981).

The glucose-tolerance test is a way of measuring the body's ability to utilize carbohydrates; diabetes mellitus is a disorder of carbohydrate metabolism. In the standard test, a blood sample it taken to determine the patients's fasting glucose level. (Glucose is the end product of carbohydrate digestion.) Then a single dose of glucose is administered, and blood and urine samples are taken at regular intervals for up to six hours. Unusually high levels of glucose may indicate diabetes.

Unfortunately, it's not widely recognized that this test is extremely "nonspecific"; it can be falsely influenced by age, inactivity, obesity, stress and drug consumption. There's also disagreement about what constitutes a normal fasting glucose level.

75

Because of the virtual revolution in the way diabetes is diagnosed, some authorities suggest that anyone diagnosed as diabetic more than three years ago should be reevaluated. Thousands of people may be spending tremendous amounts of money on treatment they don't need — all because of one dismally inaccurate medical test.

In short, Dr. Pinckney observes, "eventually, your odds get to be like Las Vegas: The more tests you get, the better your chances of coming up with a false positive and even being treated for a disease you don't have!"

On the other hand, you'd think 10 billion tests a year would improve every American's chance of *not* dying of some silent, undiagnosed disorder. Perhaps so. Yet the fact is many of these tests are not ever performed for *your* well-being.

Too Many Tests

Because of the ever-growing threat of malpractice suits, doctors openly admit they give more tests than are really medically necessary — simply to protect themselves. Juries, historically, are more inclined to believe a doctor who ordered an additional diagnostic test rather than one who relied on his clinical judgement that the test wasn't necessary.

As a result, three out of every four doctors polled by the American Medical Association in 1977 admitted they practice "defensive medicine" — ordering extra tests as protection against potential lawsuits. Over half said they ordered one or two extra tests; a quarter said they ordered three or four; and one in ten admitted they were ordering five or six additional tests. Not surprisingly, 76 percent of the doctors said their patients' medical bills were going up because of this practice (*American Medical News,* March 28, 1977).

Two other reasons for the astounding growth of medical testing that have little or nothing to do with your health: It's extremely profitable for doctors to do blood and urine tests in their own offices. An article in a recent medical journal described how a physician could add $60,000 to his annual earnings by doing his own testing. Medical tests are also ordered as part of "routine" admissions procedures at hospitals (even if they've already been done), or by schools, employers or government agencies. In other words, they may not be ordered for your benefit as much as they are for the convenience and profit of institutions.

Ignoring Abnormal Results

But perhaps the most remarkable wrinkle in this story is the evidence that this $140 billion worth of medical tests rarely changes a diagnosis or course of treatment anyway—even when the test results show some abnormality. One British study examined the use of lab tests in the management of 174 patients admitted to hospitals as medical emergencies. The researchers tried to rank all the tests that were ordered on the basis of "value of cost" by assessing the number of actions taken in the care of the patient compared with the cost of the test. Of all the routine blood and other biochemical tests ordered, only 2 percent resulted in any change in treatment at all. Chest x-rays (the highest-ranked) resulted in some action 18 percent of the time.

"There can be little doubt that many tests are requested thoughtlessly," the researchers conclude. "One hundred and ninety-two tests were requested diagnostically ... upon which no action was taken. It is difficult to avoid the conclusion that these investigations were a waste of resources" (*Annals of Clinical Biochemistry*, November, 1980).

These tests may be requested "thoughtlessly," or their results may simply be ignored or discounted. In another study, researchers at the University of Nebraska Hospital noticed a considerable number of cases where doctors did not respond to lab test results showing low hemoglobin (anemia) in their patients. So, for three months, they tried prominently marking abnormal test results with a questionnaire requesting some response from the physician. But it didn't seem to do any good. "We could find no effect of the chart reminders on the number of cases in which an abnormal admission hemoglobin value was overlooked or ignored," the researchers noted. With or without the "chart reminders," about 16 percent of the abnormal test results were disregarded by doctors (*Journal of the American Medical Association*, May 1, 1981).

So what's to be done about all this? If medical tests can be riddled with error, and doctors may ignore them anyway, should you refuse to ever submit to one again? No, but perhaps you'll be able to put the results of these tests in better perspective. "Once you're aware that most medical tests are not absolutely reliable, you are well on your way to understanding test results the way your doctor does," Dr. Pinckney says. Adds former *New England Journal of Medicine* editor Franz J.

Ingelfinger, M.D., "The capabilities of medicine, great as they are, have been oversold." Medical test results are not God's truth, they're more like probabilities; and the doctors who use them are no closer to being gods themselves than anybody else.

But, though medical testing may be imperfect, it always costs money and nearly always involves some risk, even it it's only a needle in your arm. That's one of several things Dr. Pinckney would like patients to remember. "All tests involve some risk, and that's not something you should take lightly," he told us. "Ask questions; find out about the risks. You should also remember that test results are only one small part of what a doctor uses to make a diagnosis. They're just a tool.

"But most important, I'd like patients to ask two questions. First, 'If the results of this test are positive, will it change treatment?' And second, 'If the results of this test are negative, will it change my treatment?' If both answers are no, why have the test?"

Another simple rule: "Never under any circumstances, rely upon the good or bad results of a single medical test."

Actually, there are ways you can participate in your own diagnosis and help ensure the accuracy of medical tests. You should fully inform your physician about factors that might affect test results: More than 60 tests are distorted if you're taking oral contraceptives, for example, and vitamin E can alter the results of blood and hormone tests. You should also inform yourself about the nature, risks and accuracy of tests, by asking questions or reading books like the Pinckney's encyclopedia.

You might even consider taking the stethoscope in your own hands and doing the testing yourself. Over 150 "do-it-yourself" medical tests are now commercially available, from pregnancy tests to those for urinary-tract infections and bowel cancer. Some, like blood-pressure readings, have been shown to be much more accurate when you take them yourself in the quiet of your own home.

If you *do* request the services of modern medicine, don't forget what you've learned about its shortcomings—and don't give up your right to question, to understand and to decide. It is, after all, your life, your body and your health.

CHAPTER 14

Unsuspected Medical Blunders

The infamous surgical sponge misplaced in someone's abdomen during an operation, the doctor who hands down the prognosis of "terminal" to a perfectly healthy person, the surgeon who cuts the correct organ but the wrong patient—these are the popular stereotypes of the medical mishap. They're one-in-a-million foul-ups that draw grins and shudders—and often accompany the false impression that medical bobbles are uncommon as comets.

Actually there are plenty of not-so-rare miscues to leave us wondering. It wasn't that long ago that doctors were routinely removing patients' large bowels to treat epilepsy, freezing stomachs to cure peptic ulcers and cutting out adrenal glands to lower blood pressure. All of which had about the same cure rate as eye of newt and toe of frog. Somebody goofed. And there's every reason to believe that there's a good deal of goofing still going on.

As proof of that fact, we present the following catalog of little-known slipups. It's a reminder that medical people are just like us—fallible. And that's the best argument there is for approaching professional health care with a critical eye and a questioning mind.

Ignoring the Anesthetized Patient

You're right in the middle of open-heart surgery. You're under general anesthesia, and your surgeon has just opened up your aorta. Suddenly he says, "This patient's chances are awful. There's too much damage here."

Can you, in your anesthetized state, hear his terrifying declaration? And if so, is hearing it likely to do you any harm? The pat answer from your surgeon would probably be no on both counts. But there's a growing body of evidence that suggests the pat answer isn't good enough any more.

"Surgeons are taught that because patients can't recall anything that happened while they were under general anesthesia, they can't hear anything either," says Henry L. Bennett, Ph.D., of the University of California, Davis, School of Medicine. "But the patients' amnesia is no guarantee that they weren't affected by conversations that took place in the operating room."

To prove that point, Dr. Bennett and his colleagues devised a unique experiment. They selected 32 patients scheduled for surgery requiring general anesthesia, then divided them into two groups. During surgery both groups received about the same level of anesthesia but were exposed to very different sounds. The control group encountered only the normal noise and conversation of the operating room. But the experimental group got a sound track loaded with reassuring words, pleasant music and brief instructions to touch their ears when they talked to an interviewer after surgery.

Sure enough, the experimental group later touched their ears significantly more than did the control group—even though they couldn't recall getting any suggestion at all on the operating table.

"Surgical patients under general anesthesia can be influenced by what's said in the operating room," Dr. Bennett says. "And that means they may be affected by negative statements regarding their health made during surgery. I think doctors and nurses are unaware of the effect every time they talk in surgery as though their anesthetized patients weren't there."

Making Bad Penmanship a Health Hazard

One patient mistakenly gets Maalox every hour instead of every night. Another gets ten tablets of Lasix per day instead of the proper dose of one tablet daily. Someone else takes an overdose of 1,000 milligrams of Cytoxan instead of 100 milligrams. Are these pharmaceutical faux pas the work of careless patients or drunken druggists? No, just doctors with rotten penmanship. These actual medication errors were caused by illegible prescription writing. The renowned physician's scrawl— the scribbling you thought every pharmacist could correctly decode—is a far bigger health hazard than you might have imagined.

Recently 50.9 percent of the pharmacists responding to a questionnaire published in *American Druggist* admitted making errors in dispensing because of doctor's sloppy handwriting. And in a study of prescription illegibility, two researchers at the Children's Orthopedic Hospital and Medical Center in Seattle recorded dozens of interpretation errors when medical people tried to decipher typically garbled prescriptions. Fifty people, including pharmacists and pharmacy students, read 105 actual prescriptions—and *mis*read them about 30 percent of the time (*Veterinary and Human Toxicology,* February, 1980).

Says one of the researchers, William O. Robertson, M.D., "The readers spent an average of 14 seconds on each prescription and still made far more errors than they should have. Obviously, illegibility of prescriptions can have an enormous impact."

But can you do anything to protect yourself against your doctor's scribbles? Dr. Robertson thinks so. "You would do well to ask your physician the name and dosage of your prescribed medication," he says. "Then you can compare that information with the label on the medication container. You might also check the code imprint—the numbers or letters often stamped on tablets and capsules. The imprint identifies specific medication and should generally be the same each time you get a prescription refilled. If it's different, ask your pharmacist about it."

Botching Blood-Pressure Screenings

Has your doctor diagnosed you as hypertensive? If so, maybe you should diagnose the diagnosis. For it's widely known in medical circles that a lot of people with normal blood pressure have been mistakingly told that their pressure is too high. Experts suggest that many mis-diagnoses arise because medical professionals fail to take into account the nonphysical factors that influence blood pressure.

Like talking, for instance. Recently James J. Lynch, Ph.D., of the University of Maryland School of Medicine, and his associates verified a clear connection between speech and both blood pressure and heart rate. They monitored the blood pressure and heart rate of 178 men and women (some hypertensive) and discovered that during speech blood pressure rose significantly in 98 percent of them, and heart rate shot up in 93 percent. Regardless of age or environment, the readings almost always jumped (*Israel Journal of Medical Science,* May, 1982).

"This pressure-speech connection is probably one of the most important factors that might contribute to sudden changes in blood pressure in a doctor's office," says Dr. Lynch. "Some people's pressure can shoot up 50 percent in 30 seconds after talking, though the average is more like 10 to 25 percent. So simply chatting with your doctor can radically alter your BP reading. And most physicians are only now aware of this."

To get around the problem, Dr. Lynch recommends measuring blood pressure several times—once while the patient is resting, once while silent and another time while talking. From the repeated readings a more accurate picture of blood pressure should emerge. The technique offers a new twist to a tried-and-true principle: To compensate for unknown influences on blood pressure, several readings are better than one.

And judging from research on misdiagnosing hypertension, the multiple readings are worth the trouble. One study suggests that being mislabeled as hypertensive may be as bad as actually *being* hypertensive. The researchers examined 71 people with normal blood pressure who were mistakenly told that their pressure was high. Compared to a correctly labeled control group with normal pressure, the mislabeled group suffered far more depression and thought themselves much less healthy. And their feelings of ill health had nothing to do with their actual health status or medical treatment (*American Journal of Public Health,* November, 1981).

Making the Wrong Call
on Mental Health

Someone you know is handed a preliminary diagnosis from his psychiatrist or family physician: functional psychosis, a serious form of mental illness. Should he get a second, more definitive opinion?

Darn right. The reason is that a surprising number of preliminary psychiatric diagnoses are frequently dead wrong. So say many behavioral experts, including Robert S. Hoffman, M.D., formerly chief of the medical/psychiatric unit at St. Mary's Hospital in San Francisco.

He studied 215 patients initially diagnosed as having behavioral disorders and discovered that 41 percent of them had been shoved into the wrong psychological pigeonhole. The error rate was slightly higher for those originally diagnosed with dementia, a mental disorder most frequently afflicting the elderly. At least 37 percent of the "demented" patients weren't demented at all, but suffered from other treatable disorders. "Unfortunately, the only psychological diagnosis many patients get is a preliminary one," says Dr. Hoffman. "Because they don't get a more rigorous evaluation, they're often left with an inaccurate assessment of their condition. The consequences can be inappropriate treatment or a lifetime in an institution."

Doctoring Long Distance

Has your physician ever tried to treat you via telephone? Sometimes such a practice makes perfect sense. Too often, though, it makes for royal snafus.

"All the bad habits of sloppy medical care converge in the still-too-common practice of diagnosing illness by phone and prescribing drugs without ever seeing the patient," says George D. LeMaitre, M.D., author of *How to Choose a Good Doctor* (Andover). "There are rare occasions when a patient may benefit from a telephone diagnosis. When, for example, a patient's chronic illness is well known to his doctor, a telephone diagnosis may save an unnecessary office visit. But in the vast majority of cases, diagnoses over the phone border on malpractice.

"A characteristic error is the misdiagnosis of a bellyache," Dr. LeMaitre says. "A patient calls in complaining about the pain three days in a row. The doctor assumes it's probably nothing serious and, by phone, prescribes a nonaspirin painkiller. The problem turns out to be a ruptured appendix."

Misreading the Pictures

If you had a bad heart, your doctor might ask you to undergo coronary angiography, the test in which x-rays are used to scrutinize the arteries and heart. And on the basis of the test results, he might schedule you for bypass surgery. Trouble is, there's an excellent chance that the results of the angiography would be as misleading as an errant road sign. A ton of research has already implicated coronary angiographies and pointed to their most significant failing: Angiographers, those who interpret the x-rays, are misinterpreting.

Jeffery M. Isner, M.D., associate professor of medicine and pathology at Tufts University, in Boston, is one of the researchers who helped uncover the incriminating evidence. He conducted a study in which three experienced angiographers examined the coronary x-rays of 28 deceased patients. When he compared the patients' autopsy reports with the angiographers' evaluation of the x-rays, he saw discrepancies everywhere. At least 64 percent of the evaluations failed to match the autopsy findings (*Circulation,* vol. 63, no. 5, 1981).

Have patients gone to surgery because somebody misinterpreted angiography x-rays? Certainly, says Dr. Isner. Which is why some experts suggest supplementing the tests with other data before rushing off to the operating room. For the patient, the possibility of error is just another reason for exercising a critical eye and questioning mind.

CHAPTER 15

All about Root-Canal Therapy

Suddenly you know you can't wait any longer. Your tooth is in pain and the whole side of your face is throbbing in response. The dentist confirms your worst fears—the nerve has died and become infected. It's root-canal therapy or lose the tooth.

It's not as if you've never heard of this procedure before. It's that you've heard too much, and none of it good. Now it's time to separate fact from fiction, time to learn for yourself—and not from somebody else's bad experience—just what to expect.

Ease up. The news is good. It's no longer a painful procedure and the success rate is high—about 94 percent.

But you need to know much more than that to ease your mind. That's where we come in. Out list of questions and answers covers all aspects of the procedure, including potential complications (yes, there are a few rare ones).

To help us we went to the experts, the dentists who specialize in root-canal therapy, called endodontists. Donald Arens, D.D.S., is an associate professor at the Indiana University School of Dentistry, in Indianapolis, and former president of the American Association of Endodontists. Michael Heuer, D.D.S., is a professor at Northwestern University School of Dentistry, in Chicago, and vice president of the American Association of Endodontists. And Irwin Smigel, D.D.S., a general dentist, is author of *Dental Health, Dental Beauty* (M. Evans) and a postgraduate lecturer at the New York University College of Dentistry.

Q: What exactly is root-canal therapy?

A: It's the complete removal of a tooth's nerve. That means the part that not only fills the hollow center of every tooth (crown), but also the parts that continue as canals down into the root below the gum. The nerve is removed when it has died and become infected.

Q: What causes the nerve to die?

A: Most often it's from a neglected cavity. Once decay has penetrated the dentin (the layer under the enamel) it can move on to the pulp (the center of the tooth, which contains the nerves and blood vessels). Now the nerve is exposed to germs and infection can set in, causing an inflammation and swelling inside the canal. Since the root canal is rigid, this swelling strangles the pulp, cuts off its blood supply and kills it.

A trauma to the tooth, such as a severe blow, or even excessive heat from a drill, can also cause irreversible nerve damage. If blood flow (and the oxygen it carries) to the nerve is interrupted, the nerve begins to die. Dr. Smigel compares it to stroke victims whose oxygen to the brain is temporarily cut off. Brain cells die, often leaving permanent damage, just like the nerve of a tooth.

Q: Why does the tooth hurt if the nerve is dead?

A: A nerve that has died almost always becomes abscessed. Eventually the gases that build up inside the canal burst through the bottom of the root, deep in the gum, spreading infection and pus to surrounding areas. While the dead nerve *inside* the canal is no longer causing pain, the nerves in the jawbone and in the *outer* covering of the root (cementum) are still alive—and surely let you know it.

Q: Can I have a dead nerve without pain?

A: Yes. While the nerve is dying, there is usually a great deal of pain. But it disappears completely after the nerve has died. It's actually possible to go years without further trouble—but it's unlikely. That's because bacteria love to munch on the dead pulp and sooner or later (usually sooner) it will abscess.

Q: How can a dentist be sure that my problem is caused by a dying or dead nerve?

A: The dentist will conduct a few very simple tests on the tooth in question as well as the teeth surrounding the "bad" one. First he will see how your teeth respond to heat, then cold, and finally to an electrical pulp tester that sends a low current through the tooth.

In a normal, healthy tooth, you should be able to feel the heat, cold and electrical current as clearly uncomfortable—meaning the tooth is alive and well. Of course the dentist stops as soon as you signal that you've felt it. Then the discomfort should stop immediately, too.

All normal teeth should respond similarly, so that a tooth that doesn't becomes suspect. For example, a tooth whose nerve is in the process of dying shows a lower level of current. Ice causes pain that persists after it's removed and then gradually goes away. Heat, on the other hand, causes a *severe* toothache that can actually be relieved by something cold.

If the nerve is completely dead, you will not feel anything at all when the tooth is tested.

"These tests are very valuable," says Dr. Heuer, "but they are not foolproof. I'd say they're about 75 to 80 percent accurate, so it's important to your dentist to use other diagnostic tools as well. Is there a deep filling? Has there been a trauma to the tooth? What does the x-ray show? Has there been pain on previous occasions? Then he will be better able to make a correct diagnosis."

Q: When the pulp (nerve) is removed, is the tooth dead?

A: As Dr. Heuer likes to point out, "No tooth is dead until you've got it in your hand." Sure, the internal organ (pulp) is gone, but there are still nerves and blood vessels feeding the outside of the tooth—the cementum and periodontal ligament.

Q: Is root-canal therapy painful?

A: No. In most cases the procedure can be done painlessly. A dentist can numb the area with novocaine, so that you will feel the pressure of the instruments but no pain. Once the numbness wears off there may be some discomfort for a day or two due to inflammation in the periodontal ligament at the root tip created by working on the tooth.

Q: How is root-canal therapy done?

A: Very carefully. The dentist uses a mechanical drill only to clean out the nerve in the crown of the tooth, but then uses hand instruments for the rest of the procedure. These instruments, called reamers and broaches, range in size from tiny to tinier, depending on the size of the canal they must be inserted into. By twisting and thrusting these instruments into the canal, the dentist is able to remove all of its contents. Meanwhile, the canals are continuously flushed to remove debris. After that the canals are smoothed and shaped with special files to prepare them for the filling material.

The preferred filling, Dr. Smigel told us, is gutta-percha, a natural rubberlike substance derived from the sap of a tropical tree. It shapes itself to fit the inside of the canal and seals off the tip of the root completely. It can also be easily removed if the root canal has to be reworked for some reason.

The other material that is sometimes used is silver point filling. But this is "difficult, if not impossible," to remove once it's in place, and it doesn't create as good a seal, explains Dr. Smigel.

Q: How does the dentist know if he has filled all the canals in a tooth?

A: It's tricky, all right. Because even though certain teeth have a particular number of roots (from one to three, depending on the tooth) a root may actually have *more than one canal.* And every one must be cleaned thoroughly to the bottom and then filled. Since the dentist is working in the dark (so to speak), he must rely on precision instruments and x-rays to see if he's reached the bottom.

Q: How many visits to the dentists does it take to complete the root-canal therapy?

A: Usually three. The roots are completely cleaned out and sterilized on the first visit. A temporary filling is put in, but sometimes an opening is left for drainage if the infection is severe.

The second appointment seems a lot like the first, but actually the dentist is cleaning the canals even more thoroughly and is shaping them in preparation for the filling.

At the third and final visit, the dentist puts in the gutta-percha filling.

Q: Why do the root canals have to be filled?

A: "It's the old story of 'Nature abhors a vacuum,' " Dr. Smigel points out. "If the dentist doesn't fill the canals after the nerve has been removed, the body will fill them itself—with bacteria."

It's also part of what Dr. Arens calls "the triad of success. Get to the bottom of the root, clean it out completely and make it solid to keep out the germs."

Q: Can root-canal therapy be done successfully on any tooth?

A: No. Some teeth have roots that are so crooked or so narrow that inserting the reamers to the bottom is virtually impossible. And cleaning out only the part of the root that can be reached will never do. Any nerve material left inside becomes the next main course for bacteria.

Also, the roots of very old teeth sometimes become calcified and so hardened that even a hammer and chisel won't budge them.

Even when root-canal therapy can be completed (which is most of the time), there is still a slight chance that it won't correct the problem.

Q: What can be done next, short of losing the tooth?

A: When infection persists despite completion of the root canal therapy (pain will tell you something is wrong), your dentist may recommend a procedure called an apicoectomy, which is done by an endodontist or oral surgeon. The still-infected roots are approached by cutting through the gum and bone between the root and cheek. The surgeon exposes the root, cleans out the infection and sometimes cuts off the tips of the infected roots to make sure the source of the infection is gone—permanently. The ends of the roots are then sealed off with a filling material.

For people whose roots are too crooked, too narrow or have become calcified, there is yet another option, says Dr. Arens. "We can extract the problem tooth, clean and seal the roots and then replant it in the mouth—all within 30 minutes. A temporary splint is required to hold it in place," explains Dr. Arens. "The success rate is 80 percent, not quite as high as conventional root-canal therapy, but it's better than losing the tooth."

Q: What are the potential risks or complications associated with root-canal therapy?

A: If not done with attention to the infection, the dentist could make it worse, Dr. Heuer says. "It's important for the reamers not to puncture the side of the root or go beyond the apex. This could actually spread the infection."

Also, a tooth that has lost its blood and nutrient supply is more brittle and more subject to fractures. When fractures do occur, the tooth generally breaks horizontally, leaving little or no crown. But the situation isn't hopeless, says Dr. Smigel. "The remaining root can be built up with a special stainless-steel post to support a crown replacement."

Q: How much does root-canal therapy cost?

A: It varies depending on the tooth involved. After all, much more work is required in a tooth with three roots than in a tooth with just one. The cost can also vary depending on what part of the country you live in. Generally you can figure on about $175 for the simplest case to about $500 for a more complex problem. To be sure, ask your own dentist.

It's likely, however, that pulling the tooth and replacing it with a false tooth or bridge would be far more expensive.

Q: What is the life-span of a tooth that has been through root-canal therapy?

A: Barring any unforeseen complications, there is no reason why the tooth shouldn't last as long as any of your other "normal" teeth, our experts told us.

"Root-canal therapy has always had a worse reputation than it deserves," says Dr. Heuer. "But with the refinements of existing techniques, your chances are better than ever for a successful outcome."

Rodale Press, Inc., publishes PREVENTION®, the better health magazine.
For information on how to order your subscription,
write to PREVENTION®, Emmaus, PA 18049.